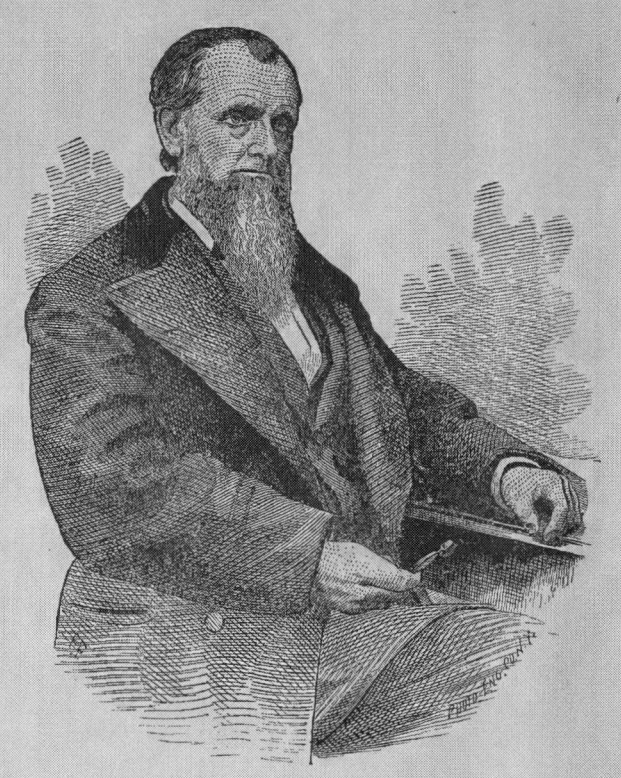

GEO. F. ADAMS, M. D.

TURKISH BATH

HAND BOOK,

EDITED AND COMPILED BY

GEO. F. ADAMS, M. D.

ST. LOUIS, MO.

For the distant still thou yearnest,
And behold the good so near!
If to use the good thou learnest,
Thou wilt surely find it here.

—GOETHE.

1881.

LITTLE & BECKER, ST. LOUIS.

CONTENTS.

PREFACE.

"However plausible," says Dr. Shepard,* "may be the theories which relate to treatment of disease, and however sanguine may be the views of enthusiastic specialists, they have no practical significance in this practical age, if they are not sustained by experimental facts and elucidated by impartial inquiry."

It is to the elucidation of the merits of the "Turkish Bath" by impartial inquiry and experimental facts that I now offer to my friends and the public generally this Hand Book on Turkish Baths. I have compiled the following pages from the best authorities, and spared no pains to get at facts,—*no theories, no romancing.*

It is not generally known by the public that there is scarcely a medical text book, published of late years, on Therapeutics, in which more or less of its pages are not devoted to the Hot Air Bath as a remedial agent in disease. Hence, the Turkish Bath is legitimatised. Surely the world moves! I hope the following pages will be read by all who take an interest in whatever tends to better the condition of our fellow creatures, for without good health life is not worth living.

The future of the Bath is full of promise, and pregnant with blessings to suffering humanity. The proved results warrant the opinion that we have, as yet, only witnessed the dawn, as it were, of a more brilliant and

---

* Physician to the Queen's household.

successful future. I may not live to see it, but trust I shall leave those to come after me, who will rejoice to see it in its full fruition.

There is pleasure in believing that among the rising generation of practitioners, there is a disposition to escape from the blind obedience hitherto exacted by established medical dogmas and medical ethics. A spirit of free inquiry is at work to test all systems by their ascertained results, and the very changes that are perpetually occurring in medical practice is the best evidence of the fact that the old faith, in its *assumed* virtues, has been badly shaken. There is a growing conviction that the whole system of drug medication is repugnant to nature,—that we cannot atone for violating the laws of life by the swallowing of drastic drugs and that such ideas are demonstrably false,—that it is essentially wrong in theory, and remorselessly destructive in practice. In conclusion (I quote another's words,) "it may be affirmed that the Turkish Bath amounts to a discovery! It is, at least, a new found boon to the States of the Western world." We claim for it to become a permanent institution among them as a remedy for most of the evils of modern civilization, —a remedy near at hand—safe, effective and agreeable. The questions it stirs are those which, next to morality and religion, intimately affect a nation's best interests. The habits it promotes are those which most directly conduce to the health, the happiness, the longevity, the physical culture, the material prosperity, and the moral elevation of the people:

It is not to be expected that objections to the bath will be suddenly overcome, or that, when ashamed to give open expression to them, the "subtle seniors" of the profession will be less active in carrying on their opposition in private, to the great detriment of patients who consider they can safely repose confidence in the rectitude and soundness of such advisers. The progress of the Bath will be in proportion to the intelligence of the public, and every year is accumulating a mass of authoritative evidence in its favor. The practictioner who disparages the bath without studying its properties or testing its merits, only exposes his incapability —his own unfitness to be trusted with the care of what is so valuable to mankind—sound health. I bear no malice toward any one, but I have written what I have written, that he who runs may read.

GEO. F. ADAMS, M. D.

Introductory Remarks.

THE CASE STATED.

Air and water are natural elements indispensable to the existence of animal life. It is not surprising, therefore, that, when modified in a greater or less degree by another natural element—temperature,—they should become the most general and powerful, the most salutary and unfailing agents yet discovered, for the sustentation of normal life, and the correction or alleviation of those numerous derangements to which it is exposed. No new principle is announced, no novel theory propounded; support is claimed for no speculative system; on the contrary, the only desire is to bring, in simple detail, before the public what has been known, though imperfectly practiced, for thousands of years in every quarter of the globe, but which, in our own day, despite various discouragements, has happily received scientific and practical development.

Normal life is health, and what subject rightly considered, is fraught with more vital import to thoughtful minds than the consideration of the most effectual means by which health can be preserved? "The first wealth is health,"—it is the richest inheritance with which man can be endowed, for success in life, to say nothing of the rational enjoyments of existence, is mainly dependent on its possession.

Surely, then, whatever tends to sustain or confer so great a blessing as health, ought to possess a primary value in the estimation of every intelligent being.

Physical health is physiologically necessary to perfect mental health, and this incontestible truth ought never to be lost sight of, for as Dr. Mulligan* observes, " The sound operation of the mind is frequently disturbed by the slightest physical influence."

Two schools of medicine, famous in their day, were distinguished by opposite views on this subject. Stahl, the founder of one, contended that bodily disease principally proceeded from affections of the mind, while Hoffman, the founder of the other, maintained that the primary cause of all disease was referable to the body. A more enlightened physiologist, however, now admits that there is much truth in both theories, and has established the existence of a reciprocity of action between the mental and physical which is an inflexible law of our economy, the effects of which are not speculative but demonstrative, though *how* the mysterious relationship exists and acts, is inscrutible and inexplicable. It is sufficient for all practical purposes to know that such a relationship does exist, and that health is governed by certain laws which are, in the main, well defined and easily understood. This being the case it follows that there is a moral obligation on every one who has intelligence and opportunity, to become acquainted with the laws, and live in obedience to them.

" Know Thyself," is an ancient and wise maxim, which comprehends a philosophy that lies at the root of human happiness and well being.. Next in import-

* The Passions of Mind and Matter.

ance to a knowledge of the means by which health can best be preserved, is an acquaintance with those simple and natural agencies by the judicious application of which deviation from the healthy standard can be corrected, and the balance of disordered functions re-adjusted and restored.

This knowledge, however, few persons care to acquire, the mass—even of the "educated classes"— being content to remain ignorant of those physiological laws which are the real foundation of all that is rational in medicine,—of all that has solid pretensions to rank as Hygienic, Prophylactic and Therapeutic,— that is of all which can be truly deemed preservative of health, or possessed of remedial properties in relation to the numerous derangements to which our artificial habits of life render us more or less liable.

It is within the scope of every ones observation that on such subjects deplorable ignorance prevails. How few are to be found who have rational ideas respecting their own organism,—who understand even the language of physiology, or could give a satisfactory answer to the questions, What is health? What is disease? It is, in truth, *unduly* complimentary to speak of an "educated laity" in relation to this subject, because, in reality, ignorance, and not knowledge, is the prevailing rule. Now I ask the candid reader, is not my assertion true? Yet what passes current in society for an "accomplished education" embraces at least a smattering of almost every subject, save *A knowledge of man, of his organism, his functions, and the laws that govern them.* This admitted defect in our general educational curriculum sadly tends to foster the superstitions and impositions which have for ages existed in relation to the alleged curative effect of drugs, and in this way becomes the source of an incalculable amount of human misery. The errors of one generation are thus transmitted as a baneful inheritance to another, and inveterate prejudices are perpetuated to stifle the voice of nature and of truth.

If the so-called "educated classes" really possessed such easily acquired knowledge as I have referred to, it is not possible to believe that the vocation of quackery, whether orthodox or heterodox, legitimate or illegitimate, licensed or unlicensed, would continue to be the prosperous business it has always proved, and never more so than in our own time, because it is owing to the ignorance and consequent *credulity* of mankind, that quackery in medicine finds profitable existence. "Man," observes some one, "is a dupable animal." Quacks in medicine, quacks in religion and quacks in politics know this and act upon that knowledge. Quacks in religion or politics are bad enough, but there are always corrective influences more or less powerfully at work to counteract their mischief; whereas, quacks in medicine labor in a field peculiarly their own. They appeal to the ignorance of their patients, and act on the infirmities of human nature when their seductive devices have greatest potency,— when the body is suffering from the torments of disease, and the intellect is obscured by apprehensions of fatal consequences, and hence the remarkable success which has attended empiricism, even among the best educated classes, in all ages.

How is this matter to be righted? for no one that has the smallest amount of common sense can deny the soft impeachment. The profession never will bring about the reform so devoutly to be wished for. They have been on trial for two thousand years and more. Dr. C. Kidd says: " Our chiefest hopes at present exist in the outer educated public. It is a sad but humiliating confession." Sylvester Graham says: "*Our only hope is to enlighten the public in the laws of life and health.*"

A public so enlightened would not long be retained in the bondaged drug superstition, nor be deterred by the mere *ipsedixit* of ignorance, prejudice and selfish interests from adopting remedial agencies in accordance with nature and reason.

But in order to comprehend clearly the various agencies brought to bear against the use of the Hot Air Bath by the medical faculty, it is necessary to candidly examine the state of the medical profession as it now exists, and in doing so, reliance can be most satisfactorily reposed in the conscientious expression of opinion by medical men themselves. All the conclusions arrived at in the following pages will be fully sustained by unquestionable professional authorities.

The Physiological Basis

—OF—

THE TURKISH BATH,

—BY—

John Balbirnie, A. M. M. D.,

OF LONDON.

Preface to the First Edition.

The question which we here feebly essay to expound is something more, and higher far, than the introduction amongst us of an oriental luxury, a pure custom, or new mode of cleanliness, all important as it is admitted to be, even in these subordinate points of view. THE TURKISH BATH IS A MIGHTY AGENCY FOR THE PREVENTION AND CURE OF DISEASE. It is a long sought *desideratum* of practical medicine, and will be hailed by all physiologists and physicians (who have more at heart the interests of humanity than the gains of a calling) as one of the most potent *modifiers of the living organism*, whether in health or disease. In this aspect of the subject, the more this new ally of the healing art is tested, the more it will be trusted,—the more will it vindicate its pretensions to be placed in the arsenal of physic, as an *orthodox weapon* of medical warfare. As such we believe the day will come when its machinery will be established as an integral and essential part of the equipment of every hospital, dispensary, asylum, workhouse, barracks and camp— yea, even of every public school of every civilized State. Increasing experience is bringing forth new facts every day to prove its curative powers.

Will our palaces and metropolitan club houses be long without the Bath? We trow not. How long will it be 'ere it becomes the health preserving implement of every complete private mansion? No other agency will so neutralize the drawbacks and discomforts and dangers of our cold, damp, variable climate during at least seven months in the year. Whatever may be alleged of the *curative* powers of the Bath, it can not fail, bye and bye, firmly to establish itself in the public confidence, as the grand PROPHYLACTIC of disease—the PREVENTIVE agent *par excellence*.

There can be no question but that the Turkish Bath, extensively put within the reach of the poor, will do much to supplant the baneful fascination, and to substitute the injurious stimulation of alcoholic liquors. It will become, perhaps, the most powerful antagonistic or counteractive agent the Temperance Cause has yet wielded. That sacred cause must seek, as its three grand allies in exalting debased humanity, Cleanliness, Health and Religion—and *the accredited ministers of those agencies.* The most speedy and summary way to put down the nuisance and demoralization of the GIN PALACE will be to *pit it against and to pitch against it* a Turkish Bath of at least equal decorative attractions —and offering to the poor, for the price of the poisonous dram, two hours' oblivion of their care and misery, with improved health, quiet nerves, natural appetites, and, perhaps, washed raiment at the conclusion of the process. A soup kitchen or a working man's refreshment room will be a necessary appendage to all such establishments. It will require no gift of prophecy to predict which place of resort shall receive most patronage, and how far the improved feelings and thoughts and habits so induced will pave the way for the labors of the city missionary! Will not some wealthy philanthrophist, or society of philanthrophists, try the experiment? Will not the teetotallers take up this question?

It is, perhaps not out of place here to allude to, to demolish a prevalent misapprehension on the subject of the Turkish Bath: it is supposed to be only suitable for strong constitutions! This is a complete mistake. The weakly, to the contrary, as they have more need for it, are, perhaps, more benefitted by it. Its influence as an instrument of *training*,—as a means of physical development—is the least questioned and questionable. Powerfully aiding nutrition, it manifestly promotes growth and strength. For all, therefore, in whom nutrition is depraved or defective—for the scrofulous, the consumptive, the ill-nourished, the enfeebled, the emaciated, etc., the Turkish Bath is pre-eminently adapted. Nor is any extreme of age beyond its scope. Indeed, the national use of the Bath, for ages, by the Persians, Greeks, Romans, and (since the conquest of Constantinople) by the Ottoman nations, demonstrates, at least, the utter groundlessness of its alleged dangers.

But every excellent thing, even the best, may be abused. The Turkish Bath is too powerful an agent for good not to be an equal instrument of evil *when misapplied*. Its dose requires to be regulated like that of any other remedy—and this certainly is the province of the physician. To be wielded, therefore, with safety, precision and success in the treatment of disease, and for the invigoration of the delicate—to be delivered from the evils of its maladministration, and to prevent such accidents as have already occurred in this country—to save, in short, a good cause from

— 18 —

a bad name, the Turkish Bath must be under scientific
prescription and skilled superintendence.

In conclusion, it may be affirmed that the Turkish
Bath amounts almost to a DISCOVERY! It is, at least,
a new found boon to the States of the Western World.
We claim for it to become a permanent institution
among them, as a remedy for many of the evils of modern civilization,—a remedy near at hand, safe, effective
and agreeable. The questions it stirs are those which,
next to morality and religion, intimately affect a
nation's best interests. The habits it promotes are
those which most directly conduce to the health, the
happiness, the longevity, the physical culture, the
material prosperity and the moral elevation of the
people.

JOHN BALBIRNIE.

CLAREMONT HOUSE, GREAT MALVERN, May 8, 1863.

Preface to the Second Edition.

In issuing a new edition of this essay, the Author regrets that the most of it has been worked off and stereotyped while absent on a tour. This has prevented both press corrections and the addition of new matter necessary to perfect the physiological *rationale* of the Turkish Bath. It strikes the writer that his own and all other explanations of its action and virtues have been too *mechanical*—have been founded too much on what might be termed the SCAVENGER WORK of the Bath—its *safety valve opening and drain flushing* operations. Undoubtedly this is a true and all important point of view, and *alone* would place the Turkish Bath on a high pinnacle of pre-eminence, not only as a means of cleanliness and luxury, but as an instrument of Therapeutics. To macerate the corporeal tissues, and thereby to soften and open up their porous structure, obstructed by disease, by sedentary occupations, or by luxurious modes of living; to clear off the epidermic varnish that mars the *breathing functions* of the skin, to exalt its exhalant and absorbent powers, and thereby to enhance its uses as a prime agent of the aeration and CIRCULATION, as well as of the purification of the blood; to set free the blocked up excretions of the body by clearing their eliminatory outlet, and thus to facilitate what is called "the metamorphosis of structure," by powerful, yet unweakening perspiratory drains, to equalize the distribution of the blood on the surface and in the interior, and thus to undo congestions of vital viscera. Simultaneously with all this, to *poultice* (as it were) the extremities of the nerves, to sooth the sentient external surface, thereby most effectively quelling internal irritation and quieting brain excitement ; and finally to close the patulous pores and brace the relaxed muscles ; and then virtually to *electrify* the whole system by the finishing off ablutions ; certes, these are grand ends to gain—an immense boon to the sick or the sound man ; and these, moreover, are the express aims and " indications " of all medical practice, by whatsoever name called. Thank God, the sure accomplishment of these ends is the valid boast—we had almost said the exclusive prerogative—of the Turkish Bath ! So far we can point to its *demonstrable* sphere of action. This is, however, the utmost length that writers have hitherto gone in their appreciation of the *modus operandi* of the Bath. But these effects, how valuable soever, are, after all in a sort merely *mechanical*, and constitute only one half, perhaps the least potent half, of the physiological benefits of the Bath. There is something more and greater far beyond—something "behind the scenes," though less palpable, yet paramount. We have now to unfold *vital* actions of a higher class than the results specified—actions which it is the aim of all medicines to effect ; and which the very best medicines, by a rare chance only, succeed in effecting.

That copious visible distillation of fluids from the skin has its precise counterpart and analogue in the excretory actions taking place within—on the mucous, and even from the *serous* surfaces—from the ducts,

and even the parenchyma of glands, perhaps even from
every capillary tube and strainer. In this grand interior physiological *molimen* taking place always under
the operation of the Bath, is to be sought the explanation at once of its invigorating and of its curative
powers.

As elucidating the philosophy of EXCRETION, or the
DEPURATING ECONOMY of the body—we have on page
22 referred, in brief, to the beautiful physiological
doctrine of CELL-FORMATIONS—minute vesicular bodies
wherein all the chemico-vital actions of the organism
are effected. By the growth, filling and bursting of
these nucleated cells, all absorption, all secretion, and
all nutrition are performed. We were content there
with a mere allusion to the subject; but as it constitutes in a sort the very *key of the position*—the strong-
hold of the fortress of truth—the Bath partisans contend for, the subject must be opened up at greater
length, and illustrated and enforced so far as limited
space will allow.

Both the *organizing* and the *disintegrating* acts of
secretion are examples of the beginning and ending of
the cell life now in question. The favorite conditions
for the development of cell action, when the dormant
or latent germs of it exist, are HEAT and the pure
OXYGEN of the atmosphere. Instance the case of the
growth of the chick in *ovo*, or of the seed in the soil,
even if that seed has lain 3,000 years in the coffin or
stomach of a mummy! Here *cell development* or
secretory action in the *fons et origo* of the formative
nisus, and not only the beginner, but the maintainer
and the ender of it, till the "topstone" of the animal or
vegetable structure is put on. How is all this proved?"

the unphysiological reader asks. We reply, "the microscope has brought to light these dark arcana of nature." Let this reply so far suffice for the present. No instructed medical man will think that in treading this ground I am going out of my way for material of defense of the Turkish Bath. The phenomena of the gardener's *hot-house* (whether it be in the way of developing almost at will, foliage, flowers or fruit,* *or whether in keeping in health and vigor tender exotics that our rude clime would be fatal to without such fostering care*)—I say these familiar phenomena are illustrations of our control over CELL-ACTION. The sights in our prize cattle exhibitions show our control of the SECRETORY ACTIVITY of *animal* organisms, pushed even to a *morbid* excess. The simple agents at work here, in addition to the *nutrient materials* (which must, in all cases, constitute the platform of operations), are temperature and pure air. Of course, VITAL ACTION is, above and beyond all, THE CONTROLLING POWER. But the grand point to insist upon is, that this very supreme vital action is itself under the control of Art. Those SECRET, SECRETORY, FORMATIVE PROCESSES, which we can initiate and evoke at will, as in the chick or seed, or which we can control in the animal as to produce all modifications of blood, bone, nerve, vessel, brain, muscle; or by which, in the case of plants, we vary at pleasure roots, stems, branches, leaves, buds, flowers, fruit,—these, I say, are PRECISELY THE SAME PHYSIOLOGICAL ACTIONS WE CALL POWERFULLY INTO PLAY IN THE TURKISH BATH. This has not been laid due stress upon—if the point has been mooted at all, and we are not aware that it has. A thousand facts prove that the caloric and oxygen of

the air, largely received by every pore of the skin and
every vesicle of the lungs, start into unwonted activity
the processes of *cell-development or secretory action*.
This is the basis and beginning of all salutary, life-
exalting, disease-curing efforts on the part of the
organism. Of course the subsidiary agency of diet
and regimen, air, exercise and repose, must be invoked
and scientifically regulated. But in virtue of this
secret physiological machinery of cell-operations—a
true secretory *nisus*—it is in our power often, suddenly
and at once, to extinguish the disease, and re-constitute,
re-build and re-energize the dilapidated and decaying
bodies of our fellow men,—if slowly sometimes, and
by a very bit-by-bit process—yet unfalteringly and
without failure as without check, *in the same way, by
the self-same mechanism, as the coral insect (out of its
secret infinitesimal secretions) piles up its rock-reef or
sea-girt isle*. After these palpable and pertinent instances of CELL-ACTION, who shall attempt to call
" romancing," or to think incomprehensible, incredible
or mysterious the infinitesimalism of nature's operations, or to question the grand results they achieve.
*Si le grand Dieu est grand dans les grandes choses, il
est tres-grand dans les petites.*"

Space forbids us here to persue the subject ; we have
thrown out sufficient hints for the reflective. I have
given the clue to the true *rationale* of the best results
of the Bath.

JOHN BALBIRNIE.

THE TURKISH BATH. SOUTHPORT, July 30, 1864.

THE TURKISH BATH.

CHAPTER I.

THE PHYSIOLOGICAL BASIS AND ACTION OF THE TURKISH BATH — THE PHILOSOPHY OF DEPURATION — THE PENALTIES OF NON-DEPURATION.

"THE BLOOD IS THE LIFE," as charged with the great vital STIMULI, *i. e.*, the sustainers of the movements of the animated machine, the sources of its heat, and power, and action ; as containing, on the one hand, the elements of nutrition, or the building materials of the fabric—and the fuel of the living furnace ; and on the other, the atmospheric oxygen necessary to ventilate the house we live in—to combine with the products of decomposition ; thus, in one act, by one process, supporting the combustion of the body, keeping up its heat, and effecting the removal of its waste. This waste is better understood under both its popular and its scientific name—the *excretions*, or the skimmed off impurities of the body. EXCRETION is, therefore, the depurating process of animal bodies, which we must, if possible, enable the reader fully to understand if he is to comprehend the action and appreciate the virtues of the Turkish Bath.

The mere functioning or play of organized structures, every movement, great or little, of the living
apparatus, even every act of volition, every thought and
every motion, disengages heat and dissipates it, and,
therefore, by the first laws of chemistry, must wear
down and disintegrate the mechanism piecemeal.
Hence, from its first development to its final dissolu-
tion, the body is in every atom (especially of its soft
parts) the scene of incessant, even of momentary
CHANGE—of Reproduction and Decay—of the displace-
ment of the molecules of the old and effete matter,
and their combination in new forms, in order to their
exit from the body.

The healthy properties of the living fabric are maintained only so long as a due equilibrium exists between
NUTRITION and EXCRETION, or DEPURATION ; in other
words, between *supply* and *waste*—between *income* and
expenditure of body elements—between the ASSIMILA-
TION of the new materials and the ELIMINATION or exit
of the old, worn out, or superfluous constituents of
structure.

In the outgoing rounds of the circulation (*i. e.*, by
the arteries,) the blood yields up its nutrient principles for the growth or repair of the several tissues ;
in the incoming or returning circuit, (*i. e.*, by the
veins,) it receives for removal or revivification, the
particles that have been exhausted of their vitality,
or that have served their purpose in the economy.
This corporeal *debris* (*sewage*) imparts to the blood a
dark color and poisonous properties. Hence the great
importance ever attached to keeping in good working
order the EXCRETING APPARATUS of the body. This

was the grand virtue of Old Physic (which we willingly
concede to it,) of giving minute attention to the *excretions*. The aim was right, the means faulty. Irritant
medicines *create* the anomalous excretions they were
supposed to eliminate.

Secretion and Excretion are often used as synonymous terms. They mean the same thing—literally
something *separated* from the blood for specific purposes in the living mechanism. 1st. For the preparation of the nutrient materials, as the saliva, gastric and
pancreatic juices, bile, etc. 2d. For the formation of
the solids and fluids of the body, as bone, muscle,
nerve, tendon, the serous fluids of the joints and
of the "shut sacs," the humors of the eye, tears, mucus, etc. 3d. For the straining off and outlet from
the system of all substances whose retention would be
injurious—all wasted, extraneous or superfluous matters. These latter constitute the EXCRETION PROPER.
The excretions are to be viewed as the living *waste-
pipe apparatus* for equalizing, as nearly as possible,
the availing amount of the body's reparative materials
to the degree of its wear and tear. The excreted
products of the body therefore are, or should be, equal
in amount to that of the solids and fluids ingested.*

---

* A practical reflection here. A man, if he suspects his state of health,
may thus summarily test it—take disease "by the forelock," and save himself
much after suffering, by simply asking, "Is my legitimate waste in labor or
exercise equivalent to the quantity of good things I daily consume; and are
there no *capillary obstructors* among those good things?" If the answer of
conscience, or intelligence, or experience, as to these points, is unsatisfactory, then is his "nick of time" to diminish or cut off the supplies, and to hie
him to the taking-down, swilling-out and rinsing-off process of the Turkish
Bath.

"PRINCIPIIS OBSTA: sero medicina paratur,
Cum mala per longas convaluere moras."

How many valuable lives would thus be prolonged? How much invaliding
prevented? How much medical practice superseded? Is the physician philanthrophist enough to rejoice hereat!

The DEPURATING PROCESS of animals is more essential to life than even nutrition. There is but one
apparatus or system of organs, and that comparatively
a small one, appointed for the elaboration of the food.
But many and large are the instruments appropriated
to the extrication—the *excretion*—of corporeal waste.
The LUNGS, LIVER and SKIN are set apart for the
elimination of the effete or superfluous *carbon*. The
KIDNEYS are the grand outlets for the decomposed
nitrogenous matters, and the earthy and saline materials. Every other function may be suspended for a
considerable time without involving life. We can live
for weeks without food, or with the liver "locked up ;"
and several days with the functions of the kidneys
annulled ; but we can live only two or three hours with
the skin coated over, and only a very few minutes with
respiration suspended ! Hence it is clear that the
integrity of the Eliminatory or Depurating functions
is the first want of animal life—the indispensable condition of sound health. From the same facts, as well
as from the immense extent and influence of the lungs
and skin, it is very manifest that the *grand business of*
DEPURATION *falls chiefly on these organs.*

The EXCERNENT, or DEPURATING ACTIONS and APPARA-
TUS of the living organism it behooves the lay reader
well to comprehend, if possible. In their philosophy
lies the basis of all explanations of either the Theory
or the Practice of the Healing Art. As elucidating
this question, we must here devote a sentence or two
to the subject of CELLS—the secret, retired, infinitesimal organisms, which are the true builders of all
animated structure. Every vitalizing act commences
in CELLS. Nutrition and secretion, growth and reno-

vation, are but a series of *cell* operations. Fat is thus *excerned*, separated from the blood, in its little bags (ADIPOSE TISSUE.) Glandular secretions are but the bursting and yielding up of the contents of the cells covering membranous surfaces, or lining the follicles and tubes of glands. The mucus, which coats the surface of the mucous membrane, is elaborated by *epithelium cells*. The *epidermis* (or scarf-skin) is but another form of these cells, their contents dried up and exfoliating. The cells are continually developed, cast off, and renewed from the germs supplied by the subjacent membrane. The cells of the intestinal VILLI (pile of tufts) select and separate from the contents of the alimentary canal the nutritious from the refuse matters. In like manner the CELLS of the secreting tubes, follicles, or passages of a gland (as the liver, the kidneys, etc.,) separate from the blood the effete matters it is its functions to elaborate and discharge (as bile, water, etc.) ORGANIZATION is simply the appropriation thus of the nutrient compounds floating in the blood, and their combination in the proportions necessary to produce all the diversified " tissues" or structures of the body—here bone, there brain ; here muscle, there mucus ; here nerve, there vessels, etc. This organizing process is sometimes called ASSIMILATION—a vivifying or life-giving process ; assimilation is literally making food *like to*, or part and parcel of the tissues.

From all the above, it will be clear that the presence of any unassimilable matters in the blood—substances foreign to nutrition—as drugs and other poisons, miasms, the *ova of entoza etc.*, or sheerly *the unremoved waste of the body*; in other words, RETAINED

EXCRETIONS—will risk the elements (*e. g.*, *hydatid sacs,
or cistircirci cellulosi,*) In this way worms are found
in the brain, "flukes" in the liver, etc.; cancerous
tumors are developed, and deposits of tubercle formed,
etc. In the same way we have to explain the local
irritations, the pains, the functional disturbance of organs, the deteriorated nutrition, the decline of strength,
and the constitutional suffering attending the course of
certain diseases. In short, the alterations in the body
effected by the loss of balance between the functions
of nutrition and depuration—the retention or retarded
elimination of the products of decomposition—or foreign substances accidentally or voluntarily introduced
—lie at the foundation of most diseases, and constitute
their most palpable material conditions. The mere
reactions taking place between the solids and fluids of
the body, *in channels where the circulation is barred*
(e. g , in congested viscera,) suggests, even to the lay
mind sufficient cause of deranged health, malaise and
misery. Imagine only half an inch of the finest hair—
an eye-lash—dropped in among the machinery of a
Geneva watch. The living organism is, beyond all
comparison, more nice and complex, and, at least, not
a whit less sensitive to disturbing causes !

*Healthy blood-making depends infinitely more on per-
fect depuration—that is, on the active condition of the
excretory functions—than on the abstractly nutritive
qualities of the food.* Whenever the body's *debris*, or
the matters of its decomposition, are not duly excreted,
a virtual and valid *materies morbi* remains to vitiate
the process of recomposition. The functions of supply being impaired—the fountains of corporeal renewal
being tainted—the *educts* and *products* of the assim-

ilative process must be faulty. Bad materials can only furnish bad building. Hence the commencing loss of high *condition* whenever man comes materially to infringe the Hygienic laws; when, for example, superfluous food and pernicious drinks combine, with the want of due activity of the lungs and skin (*i. e.*, with corporeal inaction,) to derange the balance between waste and supply. Even the diet may be proper as to quantity and quality, and the alimentary canal may be kept "clean;" but all will not avail to produce healthy blood or firm textures, *so long as the pulmonary and cutaneous safety-valves are obstructed or marred in* their play. Let me, however, here remark, so intimate are the connections and sympathies between the Skin, Lungs, Liver and Bowels, that, under the circumstances described, it is impossible to keep the alimentary canal "clean," even in the sense which leaves out of view the operations of digestion. Those who feed the best, in the popular acceptation of the term, are not the best nourished. An interior aliment will be turned to good account—any ungenial substance it contains will be neutralized, strained, or *burnt off*, provided the air breathed, and the exercise taken by the individual, be such as to keep up a highly active state of the grand eliminatory outlets of the body; in other words, *provided the* LUNGS *and* SKIN *have the fullest scope for the performance of their appropriate functions.*

Here it falls into place to illustrate the effects of inactive *depuratory organs*, from sedentary habits, indolent repose, and luxurious indulgences of all sorts. The structure and functions of man show that he was not by any means intended to be a sedentary animal.

Those who live the longest and enjoy the best health are invariably persons of active habits. *From the moment man becomes a civilized being, the Depurating process of his blood becomes less perfect; in other words, the grand excretory functions of the Skin, Lungs and Liver are less completely exercised. From that moment diseases of various type and class, and one large class in particular,—tubercular diseases (scrofula and consumption)—begin to show their ravages on his frame.* And the reason of this is very obvious. Man's habits and modes of life become then less conformable to the instinctive requirements of his constitution; his exercise is less frequent or less natural—either unremitting or not at all; his lungs are compelled to long periods of comparative inactivity; and his skin is equally diminished in function by loads of superfluous clothing, as well as made susceptible to every atmospheric variation by all sorts of "coddling" in warm rooms. By these and sundry other anti-hygienic influences, the *blood of the civilized man is infinitely less oxygenated than it should be.* He voluntarily debars himself of the means of carying off the effete matters of his body. When the lungs are imperfectly exercised, it is impossible for the skin to be healthily active in its duties; for the two go together, co-functionate (if we may coin a word.) Baths (of the old sort) and cleanliness were the best compensations the case admitted. But nothing—*save some such substitute as that now presented to the public in the shape of the Turkish Bath*—perfectly compensates the want of active exertion in a pure air; for nothing else can perfectly open, and keep open the body's safety-valves, or secure the perfect elimination of the corporeal waste.

But the worst of the case of the locked up excretions of the skin in particular is this, viz., *that the duty so shirked is thrown necessarily on the Lungs, Liver, Kidneys or Bowels.* Hence, *nolens, volens,* able or unable, the latter organs *are compelled to do double work!*—viz., to perform their own specific work, and to take up the superseded and suspended functions of the skin. For a time the constitution gives no indication of the injury of this supplementary labor or vicarious discharge of duty. But eventually, at the "turn of life,"—at the critical age,—in short, at the period of decliñe, the over-tasked, over-strained organs *knock under.* Nature tires, or gets deranged, in the unequal conflict. From this starting point, a chain of morbid causation gradually stretches its links round the organism, first impeding, then disabling function after function. The liver or kidneys utter their complaints with a voice that can neither be misinterpreted nor resisted. Congestion of the abdominal viscera is imminent, and blue-pill is at a premium, or diuretics or cathartics are in demand. The heart, lungs or brain show open and manifest signs of congestion, at least in embarrassment and tardiness in their operations. The individual ages rapidly. His face is tallowy or jaundiced. He is the victim of sciatica, or TIC, or gout, or rheumatism. In short, from a primarily inactive skin, aided by an over-active or over-stimulated stomach, and perhaps an over-worked or over-worried brain, the sufferer becomes prematurely old and regularly broken down—a victim of disease too generally incurable, involving the principal organs—all the product of impaired general and arrested local circulation—congestion of vital structures—and, with this state of matters, retained excretions and poisoned life-springs; all—all from the simple starting point of UNDEPURATED BLOOD! A host of evils, therefore, in their beginning perfectly subject to man's control, and within easy reach of remedy.

The most desolating, as the most universal scourge, of modern society, viz., TUBERCULAR DISEASE, has its origin in *impaired functions of the skin and lungs!* This is usually supposed to be purely and simply a disease of disordered nutrition. And so it is in all its essential elements. But the *fons mali* lies farther and deeper. Neither digestive derangements nor scanty nutrition ever, *per se*, generates this "foul fiend." Be it thoroughly well considered and remembered, it is only when impaired nutrition, or bad blood-making—whether from bad materials or bad stomach—coincides with forced inaction of the pulmonary and cutaneous functions—that is, with defective elimination of carbonic acid and lactic acid—that the dire blood taint in question, and its characteristic products are manifested. Multitudes of scrofulous and consumptive patients do not belong to the ill-fed classes, neither are they among the notoriously dyspeptic; or they only become dyspeptic in the advanced stages of the malady. On the other hand, it is a matter of familiar observation that your thorough-going dyspeptic—and his name is Legion—never becomes either scrofulous or phthisical. As a general rule he is a being who lives very much for himself, and therefore with extreme care—one who encompasses himself with the comforts of life—who eschews excesses, and who has a care to breathe pure air—who takes much exercise, who bestows much pains on the condition of his skin, giving it every advantage

of clothing, cleanliness, currying, suitable temperature
in doors, etc.   Besides, your gastric sufferer is usually
a keen man of business, or an ardent devotee of literature and science, and is not devoid of much
agreeable mental stimulation. *All these are conditions opposed to the inroads of tubercular disease!*
But let the circumstances of the case be reversed—let
the individual be ill-fed, ill-warmed, ill-housed, ill-clad,
ill-ventilated,—let him become the inmate, perhaps, of
a cellar residence, or a prison cell, with *moral*, as well
as *physical* depression, low spirits, etc., to struggle
with—and it will then be a miracle, if he do not,
sooner or later, exhibit some form of this exterminat-
ing disease.   But the morbid change in question
(*tuberculosis*) takes place, less because of the implication of the digestive organs, than because the lungs and
skin have been condemned to comparative, if not absolute inactivity.   The very sighing of the disconsolate
is an instinct to arouse the action of the lungs.   In
like manner the well-to-do classes, who have no material or ostensible miseries to borrow the disease from,
equally succumb, when blighted affections, grief, be-
reavements, disappointments, etc., deaden both heart
and head, paralyzing, in a sort, the skin and lungs, and
liver, if not limbs also. *In short, any one may become the mark and victim of tubercular disease, when
together with causes impairing the general health*, the
active play of the skin and lungs is impeded, *from any
circumstances whatever*.   The most potent of these are
checked perspiration, or unguarded exposures in variable climates, over-clothing as much as underclothing
of the skin, stooping posture, or confinement of chest
by ligature or stays, the influence of absorbing pas-

sions, etc., and most of all (in the highly favored classes who should otherwise escape the disease) inflammations, which congest or consolidate portions of the pulmonary tissues, and the treatment of which, as hitherto managed, entails weeks of wearisome confinement to the sick room ; too often in the olden time the poisoning of the system, and the ruining of the digestive organs, by the excessive use of drugs : bleeding, blistering, low diet and depletants, together with the depression of the vital powers by every other anti-hygienic influence.* We shall give for the present the apposite case of the monkeys in the Zoological Gardens of London, not a great many years ago. An elegant room was built for them. Every attention was paid as respects the quantity and quality of food. But one thing was wanting—*ventilation was entirely neglected!* In short, the functions of the *skin and lungs* were ignored. The consequence was, *they all died of tubercular disease* within a short time.

In conclusion of this part of our subject, we believe it may be laid down as an irrefragable truth, viz., that no one with perfectly acting skin and lungs becomes tuberculous; or being tuberculous, long remains without the arrest of the ravages of the disease.

LACTIC ACID is one of the products of the decomposition of the tissues, and *finds its chief outlet by the skin.* When the cutaneous function is impaired (*and this impairment, we contend, is an integral part of tubercular disease,*) the elimination of the lactic acid is attempted by other outlets, *chiefly by the bowels.*

---

* I shall illustrate all this another day in my medical histories of some distinguished victims of consumption.

Hence the prevailing acidity of the intestinal canal in scrofula and phthisis, remarked by all who have investigated that point. Hence the partial and temporary benefit of alkaline remedies in those diseases. This acidity of the *primæ viæ*, and the derangements of the alimentary canal associated with it, are most common in infants and children. Hence their greater tendency to manifest the mesenteric forms of scrofula.

We challenge refutation of this position, viz , that imperfect blood depuration (*i. e* , defective play of the lungs and skin,)*and not directly bad digestion, or faulty blood-making, is the primary source of the vitiation of the solids and fluids characteristic of scrofula and consumption.* A careful analysis of all the phenomena, and an extensive generalization of the best ascertained facts regarding the causation of these diseases, can lead the honest and dispassionate enquirer to no other conclusion. For our own part, we have devoted many long years to this research. The solemn and unalterable conviction of our understanding we have now uttered—and fearlessly, as becomes a truth-seeker. The foregoing observations, therefore, are a high plea, if they do not constitute an unanswerable argument, for the Turkish Bath to be established among us, co-extensively with the evils it is designed and fitted to grapple with.

Let us explain as briefly as possible the mischievous effects on nutrition of impairment of the functions of the lungs and skin—*i. e.*, of the want of adequate supplies of oxygen to combine with the carbonaceous waste of the body, and to effect its elimination from the system. This point of view will exalt

the utility of the Turkish Bath more highly in our es
timation than aught else. We have already shown
that oxygen is the first want of the animal economy
—a want of infinitely more importance than even food,
inasmuch as the products of decomposition demand
abstraction and exit, *momentarily* as they are formed.
Now, as the food contains large supplies of this most indispensable element (oxygen,) is it a very violent supposition, or a very improbable hypothesis, its reception
failing by the lungs and skin, that the economy, in its
pressing want of oxygen *borrows from this source of*
supply albeit at too dear an interest? or, as Liebig
would express it, *converts the elements of nutrition into*
elements of respiration! What more likely resource
what more natural, what easier, what more at hand,
than when the food is decomposed in the process
of digestion, and its elements set free, that a portion
of the oxygen of the fatty and albuminous matters
should be abstracted to supplement the deficit of that
introduced by the lungs and skin? In this way a radical vitiation of the alimentary principles would be
effected, thereby disabling them to perfect nutrition
precisely the extent to which they had been robbed of
oxygen. The tissues formed from this faulty material
would, of course, be defective or diseased in a corresponding ratio. This deteriorated albumen, *we know*,
presents in the case of tubercular subjects It will not
fibrillate like the albumen of healthy blood. It as-
sumes, instead, a granular, amorphus form—a form
unfit for the nutrition of the tissues. Chemistry will,
perhaps, tell us one day what precise things have taken
place in the atomic constitution of this deteriorated
albumen Is it a very far-fetched and unlikely con-

jecture, that it has parted with some atoms of its oxygen for indispensable depuration? In other words, to diminish the evils of an excess of uneliminated carbon in the system? Are we assuming too much in calling it *deoxydated albumen?* But we are fortunately not left in the same uncertainty as to the results to the oily principle of the loss of a portion of its oxygen. Chemistry even defines and gives a name to this deoxydated oil. It is a cholesterine—a form utterly unfit for nutrition. It abounds in tubercle! This we should expect. The liver is the appointed organ for eliminating the excess of fatty matters in the system. Cholesterine is a constituent of bile. When in excess in the economy, we have of course fatty liver. Now this fatty liver is peculiarly and pre-eminently the lesion of consumptive subjects The fat and oils of their diet go into the stomach sound. Here we find them in a degraded shape, *i. e.*, largely divested of their oxygen. What greater proof could we have of the principle we seek to establish, viz., that oxygen failing by the skin and lungs, Nature, in her dire extremity, when perfectly non-plussed, robs the food of it,—as it were, preferring that the machine be kept in play at any hazard and expense, rather than come to a stand at once—that the patient die slowly and gradually rather than suddenly. Need we wonder that blood globules made of such deoxydated materials are of low vital properties, and that in proportion as the system is compelled to use this faulty material, a progressive deterioration of the whole solids and fluids of the body takes place—to an extent, in the long run, utterly incompatible with the functions of life?

This which affords, for the first time, the true *ration-*

ale of fatty liver, for the first time also yields the explanation at once of the emaciation characteristic of tubercular disease, and also of the efficacy of cod-liver oil in checking that emaciation and mitigating the symptoms. By virtue of disabled lungs and sluggish skin, vitiated air, faulty posture of body, ligatures of waist, sedentary habits, close confinement in unwholesome chambers, breathing live-long nights an atmosphere unrenewed, and doubly tainted by the mephitic exhalations of bed, etc., etc.—oxygen having become an imperious want in the economy, not only in the food, robbed of a quota of its oxygen, but the available fatty tissues of the body are laid under contribution. Nature has, in fact, deposited fat in its areolar beds for the purpose of supplying the necessary oxygen during seasons of inactivity of the respiratory organs and skin. Instance, point-blank, hybernating animals, who commence the winter fat and awake lean. The same is the source of the waste in phthisis. Cod-liver oil, by presenting a large store-house of oxygenous supply, spares the adipose tissues, and so far is an invaluable nutrient element.*

---

* I answer two objections here: *First*—Why is the oxygen of the oil and albumen robbed, which have so small quantities of it to spare, compared with the starchy and saccharine principles of the food which abound in oxygen. I reply, that the oxygen is not readily get-at-able in the food in question, because they are hydrates of carbon, *i. e.*, combinations of water and carbon, which water would require to be decomposed before its oxygen was available. Now we have no proof that water is ever either formed or decomposed in the body. But the oxygen of the oil and albumen is more easily separated. Hence these principles suffer the robbery of it, and the consequent deterioration of their properties as nutrient principles. *Objection Second*—Is not your destination of food antagonistic to Liebeg's theory of heat-forming and blood-forming elements? I admit that it is; and I am prepared to prove, moreover, that Liebeg's theory of animal heat of the destination of food is open to fatal objections, which cannot be entered upon here. We give one example.: If carbonaceous foods were solely or chiefly for respiratory purposes, what becomes of the highly carbonaceous rice and ghee diet of the Hindoo, living often in a temperature above that of his body? How is this carbon burnt off without burning him up? Liebeg's theory totally fails to explain these points. How is rice and ghee incapable of sustaining an Esquimaux? Suffice it, then, to state my convictions, that every chemical research instituted will only confirm my position, that the oxygen of the fat of tubercular patients is appropriated as I allege it to be: that supplementarily the oil and albumen of the food of such patients are laid under contribution—are deoxydated for depurating purposes, in the defect of the perfect duty of the lungs and skin.

Finally, on this branch of our subject: No undemonstrable or as yet undemonstrated truth is clearer (to my own mind, at least,) than this, viz., that the available oxygen of the food is converted into an element of respiration or depuration whenever sufficient oxygen for the purpose is not forthcoming by the inlet of the lungs and skin, or sufficient carbon not eliminated by the same outlets. Here, then, is a grand impairer of nutrition—a new, and yet very old factor of disease, introduced to the notice of the profession. Is this not tracking to his lair a fell destroyer of the human race, who has long lain in ambush?

The practical views now suggested in connection with the Turkish Bath, when pushed to their legitimate consequences, will operate, we believe, a great revolution one day in medical treatment, and will influence for good the destinies of thousands of unborn generations! I challenge my respected medical brethren to refute the distinct proposition I lay down on this head, viz., deficient oxydation of the waste of the body lies at the foundation of most diseases—an evil aggravated in chronic disease, by the attempts of the system to compensate this defect by abstracting oxygen from the food!

Disprove this allegation who can.† Beyond all question, this infra-oxydation is the starting point of gout, of rheumatism, of diabetes, of granular kidney, of fatty degeneration, of many forms of fever, and

---

† My "party"—the "party" of the Turkish Bath—will doubtless challenge the profession to this disproof—to invalidate or substantiate my position. So important is the question practically, so much will the truth of this view advance the cause of the Turkish Bath, that I entertain strong hope that some rich partisan will make it the subject of a Prize Essay for German, French or British chemists to decide.

of some others of our gravest diseases. If so, what
is pointed out as the cure of this state of matters?
Less trust to mere drugs unquestionably; and more
attention to open and keep open the body's safety-
valves! This can always be done by the simplest natural agency. It would argue little wisdom and less
benevolence in the All-wise and All-merciful Designer
and Maker of all things, if we were obliged to go to the
wilds of Peru for a remedy to a disease caught on the
banks of the Thames, or in the meadows of the Sev-
ern. But fortunately for mortals, the "bane and antidote lie both before them." If I were asked to give a
brief and distinctive definition of the Turkish Bath, I
would say, it is that which claims the exclusive or pre-
eminent power of physiologically opening the safety-
valves of the living mechanism; or, in other words,
developing a high activity of the depurating economy
of the animal body, and so fulfilling the first grand indication for the cure of all diseases. If wielded by
courageous and skilled hands, no artificial or medicinal
system will be able to compete with it, either as
respects the quantity or quality of its cures. How
precisely adapted it is to arrest the ravages of scrofula
and consumption, all theory now declares—if facts
failed to speak. And we do anticipate and predict an
immense decline in the prevalence and mortality of
these maladies, from the time of the general establishment and patronage of the Turkish Bath among the
Western peoples—now their greatest victims. Among
the Eastern nations who use the Bath, this desolator of
European hearths is almost unknown. *Ecce omen*

CHAPTER II.

THE whole body may be considered, in one point of view, as a grand excretory apparatus. The Lungs, the Skin, the Liver, the Kidneys and the Bowels are but the more prominent organs for the elimination and out-let of the superfluous, wasted or noxious materials of the system. The first three only of these constitute the subject matter of the present exposition—giving simply so much of their anatomy and physiology as is necessary to the explanation of their functions. We begin with

1st. *The Lungs.* On this function all that is rele-vant or demanded for our popular treatise may be comprised in a very few lines ; and the briefer the more desirable, because we have much to say on the Skin and Liver—organs much more under our control, and therefore, more subject to abuse.

The largest product of the waste or transformation of the structures of the body is *carbon*. This is indi-cated by the dark color of the blood returning from the rounds of the circulation—exhausted, devital-ized, and loaded with the impurities of the body's decomposition, as well as with much of the ref-use of the materials of recomposition, chiefly carbon-aceous. The Divine Architect of our frames has taken corresponding precautions for its excretion or throwing out. The apparatus provided to this end is at once the simplest and the most comprehensive. The exclusive requisite is a membrane that shall admit the *diffusion of gases* ; in other words that shall expose the blood to the influence of the atmospheric air. This is all that is necessary to the outlet of the most poisonous elements of decay, and to the entrance of the supreme principles of vitalization. To purify is thus synonymous with to vivify. The air-cells of the lungs and the pores of the skin, are, respectively, the great contrivances for this purpose. It is the function of the lungs and of the skin to fulfil this conjoint office. Aeration of the blood is thus the first essential of life. Remove a fish from the water, and the gill-plates—its lungs—dry and cohere. Aeration of the blood is impossible. The fish necessarily dies In the earthworm, leech and other animals far down in the scale, there is nothing of the strict nature of lungs and gills. But other equally efficient means (for them) of aerating the blood are adopted. The change from venous to arterial blood is effected in small sacs or vesicles, usually placed in pairs along the back, and opening upon the surface of the body by means of pores in the skin called *spiracula, i e.,* breathing tubes. Close these spiracles, and you as effectually kill the animal, as by drying the gills you kill a fish, or, by obstructing a man's windpipe you "stop his vitals." In the earth-worm there are no fewer than 120 of these minute external openings between the segments of the body. In the leech there are only sixteen on each side.

Throughout the whole animal kingdom there is an intimate relation between the energy of the lavit func-

tions and the activity of the respiratory apparatus.
In cold-blooded reptiles, as the frog, respiration is
reduced to the very minimum; the vital functions are
correspondingly low and languid. In insects, on the
contrary, there is a large provision made for breathing.
In them we find vital action excessive—even vehement.
The common fly is reckoned to move its wings a thous-
and times in a second! Witness the activity of a
hive of angry bees, of hungry or thrifty ants, and the
large amount of heat they evolve! The quantity of
oxygen they consume far exceeds, relatively to their
size and weight, the proportion of any other living
creature. In the animals at the other—the high—end
of the scale, the blood is aerated by a minute capillary
net-work of vessels spread on the walls of the pulmonary vesicles or cells. In man it is calculated that 1,800
of these bladder-like dilatations are grouped around
the extremity of each air-tube, making in all some six
hundred millions. The larger of these tubes possess
muscular fibres, are hence contractile, and therefore
liable to spasms. Thus originates one form of asthma.
The average amount of carbon given off from the lungs
of an adult is about half-a-pound per diem.

The exhalation from the vast pulmonary surface is a
far greater agent in the circulation of the blood through
the lungs than the propulsive power of the heart.
This is incontrovertible; and this fact alone speaks
volumes in favor of the Turkish Bath.

2nd. *The Skin.* It is a low, incorrect and unworthy view of this grand organ to regard it only and
simply as a protective covering to the body. It is, in
truth, much more—a living, sensitive, breathing, ex-

haling, absorbing, excreting, eliminating membrane, of
exquisite structure and endowments. Herein many of
the prime operations of life take place. The skin
may truly be called a great appendage to the heart
and lungs, being an equal co-worker with them in the
circulation of the blood. It does for the larger or
systemic capillary circulation what the lungs do for the
smaller or *pulmonary* circulation. It not only rids the
blood of its carbon and supplies it with oxygen, but
regulates its density—evaporating its watery constituents. The skin is at once the grand drying, draining
and ventilating apparatus of the body. It is in itself
an universally expanded lung, kidney, liver, heart and
bowels. It is the greatest medium of nervous and
vascular expansion, and, therefore, the seat of thrilling sensibilities, and exquisite tactile endowments.
Altogether, the skin is an admirable piece of Design,
illustrating alike the Wisdom and the Goodness of the
Supreme Architect. On the sound condition of this
organ, as much as, if not more than that of any other,
depends the comfortable working of the living machinery. Its sympathies are intimate and universal
with every suffering member. On it are reflected *their*
ailments; and *its* derangements in turn, are sure materially to modify for the worse the play of the interior
apparatus. Herein is apparent how potent, not to say
how safe, a battery the skin presents for the reduction
of disease. In fact many acute maladies select the
skin as it were the common sewer for the running off
of morbid elements which have accumulated in the system, and which no over action by the bowels or kidneys by drugs has been of avail to eliminate. We
speak of the *sweating crisis* in fevers, for example.

The effect of leeches and blisters, and hydropathic fomentations and compresses, illustrates further the powerful sympathies of the surface with the textures and organs seated below. Everybody knows how in small-pox, scarlet fever and other eruptive diseases, *the battle is won or lost on the field of the skin*, according as its safety-valve functions rise or fall. If the interior irritation can be safely transferred to, and retained on the surface, all is well with the patient. Do we want a ready test of the state of health of any man, or woman or child, yea, even of our horses or oxen? We narrowly examine the skin! Its hues and its gloss, its roughness or its wrinkles, its sallowness or its pimples, speak a language the wise and experienced well comprehend.

The skin is the greatest excernent organ—the principle outlet of the body. It is a complete web of nerves and blood vessels; its thickly studded pores constitute the vastest system of corporeal drainage. Four times more matter is carried out of the body by the cutaneous surface every day, than by the alimentary canal. Costiveness or constipation of the skin, *i. e.*, constriction of its pores,—a locked up state of its exudations or exhalations—is, therefore, a much more serious affair than the same condition of the bowels. The latter may be "bound" with tolerable impunity for a week. A few hours arrested function in the case of the former may produce the most deadly symptoms; and if it were possible to seal up all the pores of the skin *at once*, as by an impermeable varnish, the individual would die in a few minutes! This accident nearly happened to a famous pugilist some time ago at the Royal Academy, where it was sought to take a cast of him *en masse*. We can now easily explain the sudden death of the boy who, at the rejoicings on the accession of Leo X to the papal chair, was *gilt all over*, to impersonate the age of gold.

The skin and the mucous membranes, or the inner and outer linings of the body, may be called and considered almost identical structures. Their functions are reciprocal—indeed substitutionary and convertible. Hence the intimate alliance for weal or for woe — the profound sympathies existing between them, and their sensitiveness to take on and resent each other's ails and aches. They are the great highways of traffic with the world without, and the vital domain within. Through them must pass *in* all the elements of corporeal reconstruction—the vivifying atmosphere and electricity—the pure *ether* of God's firmament around us—the nutrient elements, or food and drink, with salts, alkalies, earths, metals, etc. Through the same membranes pass *out* the corporal sewage, *debris* or waste — all that has served the purpose of animal economy. The obstructed functions of one or the other of these inner and outer investments of the body, originate the largest number of Acute Diseases; as in their permanent derangement lies the greatest source of inveterate Chronic Ailments. If we we want thoroughly to purify the blood, permanently to increase the tempeature, to enhance the reactive powers—to induce, in short, a radical renovation of the entire man, we must address ourselves *to exalt the functions of the skin!* In one grand point, however, these co-related organs differ—they borrow their chief nerves from different sources. These of the mucous membranes are *nerves of organic life*, and depend for their energy on the spinal *ganglia*, or centres of vegetative or automatic action. The sensitive nerves of the skin, on the contrary, belong to the domain of *animal life*, and derive their origin from the *cerebrospinal* centres. But the organic nerves are here interspersed also for the purposes of nutrition, and for the absorbent and exhalent functions of the skin. These nervous connections explain the exquisite morbid and healthy sensibilities of the skin and mucous membranes, as well as their intimate sympathies with each other, and with the centres of vitality—the brain and spinal marrow, the heart the lungs, the viscera of the abdomen, etc. In this way all morbid impressions are transmitted from without inward. By the same mechanism, the cutaneous functions in their turn become deranged by sympathy with every internal irritation; according to the extent and intensity of the interior derangment, or visceral disorder, is the healthy action of the skin marred or prevented; becoming in turn, and reciprocally, a source of aggravation to the internal malady. All digestive derangments, for example, tell upon the skin; and conversely, all cutaneous disturbance *tells* upon the digestive organs.

The texture of the skin is divisible into three principal layers: 1st, the outer scarf-skin, or *epidermis*—a simple exudation and drying up of cells or scales, in a pavement fashion, pushed upward from the *dermis chorium* or true skin, below. The scurf of the head is an illustration of the epidermic scales. It is a truly *excrementitious* membrane, and may not inaptly be deemed and designated a sort of *protection-varnish* to the vasculo-nervous web below. But as it is constantly generated, it is not a coating *intended long to be re-*

tained! Like all the structures it is of *cell* formation. Possessed of independent, inherent power of life and growth, each cell draws to itself the fluid residuum of the colorless part of the blood, and secretes a horny matter. These cells lie layer upon layer, constituting a sort of mosaic flooring. As the deeper layers are gradually pushed outward and become seperficial, their fluid portion evaporates, and they are converted into dry, flat, extremly thin, and dense scales. The abnormal accumulation of these scales is seen in many cutaneous diseases. Now it is easy to conceive how a dense compact varnish of this sort, when accumulated beyond measure—when not periodically removed—when encrusted moreover with dirt—obstructs the vent of the pores; not even admitting the tiling or layers of scales to act as a valve, and rise with the pressure of fluid from below. In the same way it is apparent how, by soaking and scrubbing, we improve the *permeability* of the skin, and, therefore, increase its fitness both for exhalation and absorption. This horny surface-skin is principally dried albumen, with unctuous matters. Alkalies combine with these and constitute a soap, or detergent. Hence the universal use of a combination of alkalies with oil for washing purposes. 2d, the *dermis*, or skin proper, or *chorium*, is an elastic network of fine fibres or strands firmly interwoven. In the meshes of these are enclosed little bags of fat —cushions you may truly term them—a regular padding, as it were, provided by the Supreme Architect, to enable the skin to resist the compressions and contusions it is daily exposed to, as well as to fill up any irregularities of the surface. These elastic cushions, with admirable foresight and benevolence, are made to abound in the soles of the feet and palms of the hands. 3d, between the upper surface of the true skin and scarf-skin, is a separate and distinct layer of blood vessels, and nerves heaped up into little conical eminences, like tufts, or the pile of plush. They are called *papillæ*. Hence this fine sensitive nervo-vascular web is called the papillary layer. The color of the skin depends on the quality and quantity of the blood in these vessels. The circulation of those of the head, face and neck, is much under the control of the nervous system, as is manifested in the opposite effects of fear or shame. The retention of the blood in these little vessels gives the mottled livid hue of the skin when chilled, and what is familiarly known as *goose skin*— the *gorged tufts*.

Inflammation of the skin consists in persistent gorging and retardation of the blood in these *papillæ*. The *pores* of the skin are minute tubes about a quarter of an inch long, and of a spiral course. A coil of this tube constitutes the perspiratory gland. On the lines of the palms of the hands and soles of the feet these pores present visible dots, 3,000 to the square inch, equivalent to seventy feet of drainage-pipe on every square inch of the body. If all the pores were joined end to end they would form a tube twenty-eight miles long! Conceive, then, the results of checked perspiration—but a few miles of this sewage-way blocked up. Yet such obstruction is more or less the characteristic of most chronic and acute diseases In these cases the excreting functions of the skin are more or less at fault. It is either scurfy, dry, and bruning, as in certain fevers and inflammations; or it is pale and dead, and parchment-like, as in long-standing digestive derangements.

To compensate this interrupted function of the skin, the liver, the lungs, the kidneys, or the bowels, assume often a vicarious or supplementary activity—a sort of double safety-valve work. Under this double duty they are very apt to break down—being then unfitted either for their own or their supernumerary functions. Hence the gravest diseases are engendered. Here drug$_s$ are but too often a powerless resource, because a fund of life, hard to replenish, has been drawn upon, which only the *organic energies*, by repose and diet, and regimen, bathing, and perspiration, etc.—all judiciously handled—can gradually restore. Hence the virtue of the Turkish Bath.

The amount of visible perspiration, as every one knows, varies with the exertion undergone, and the heat of the weather. The insensible perspiration, however, or the vapor exhaled from the skin, is a more uniform quantity—averaging from two to two and a quarter pounds per diem.*

From all this showing, then, of the nature and functions of the skin, it will at once appear how pre-eminently fitted it is, if not intended, to be the battle-

---

* The skin abounds in oil glands and tubes, analagons to the perspiratory. The unctuous secretion takes place most manifestly on the shoulders, on the face and nose, along the ridge of the eyelids, in the ear passages, and the roots of the hairy scalp. This oily product is sometimes arrested in its minute secretory tubes when the skin is either torpid or inflamed. The contents become solidified and impacted in the tubes. The projecting points get blackened with dirt or dust. When the tube is forcibly emptied an animalcule resembling a wood-louse is found imbedded in the little worm-like mould of the tube. The disease is called *acne;* vulgarly, "grog-blossoms." The uses of this oily matter are evidently to lubricate the skin, to impede its too rapid evaporation, to neutralize the soaking, relaxing effect of moisture, and to protect it against acrid substances. In the eyelids it evidently serves the purpose of a gutter, or eaves, to confine the tears and moisture of the eye. It keeps the cartilaginous cavities of the nose soft, and, with the hairs, serves to repel the intrusion of insects.

ground of the physician in his conflict with disease:
1st, from its being the seat of thrilling sensibilities—
as, in a sort, an electric surface—it is the great medium
of transmitting soothing or stimulating impressions to
the brain and spinal cord, on the one hand, and to the
viscera of the chest and abdomen on the other. The
nerves may well be compared to a system of infinite
connecting wires, or telegraph lines, along which inti-
mations of every kind are transmitted to the extremities, and all intermediate parts, and back again from
the extremities, etc., to the centres of power 2d, from
its immense superficies—consisting in the largest drain
or waste-pipe of the body. 3d, and lastly, from its
being an organ both everywhere patent to observation,
and capable, without injury, of standing a little rough
treatment when necessary.

But a still more interesting point of view of the
functions of the *skin* than even anything embraced in
these comprehensive details remains now to be developed. *Depuration*, of which (as we have seen) it is a
principal organ, is very grand work, and takes the pre-
cedence even of nutrition in the rank of importance to
life. But the highest, the first, the most indispensable
function of animals, the skin shares in common with
the heart and lungs. It justly boasts of being a
coadjutor with them in the prime faculty of *circulating
the blood. Without cutaneous exhalation there could be
no motion of the fluids!* The vital current would come
to an almost instantaneous stand. So that, however
great our admiration may be of the economy of the
skin, as the chief eliminator of the carbon and lactic
acids of the system, our ideas of its supreme utility and
importance will rise still higher, when we view it as an

organ quite as essential as either the heart or lungs to the circulation of the blood. This is a point of view many are not prepared for. Nevertheless it is the truth. It is ground that, so far as we know, has not yet been occupied by the expounders of this "Oriental question:" and it is, moreover, ground that is decisive. On this alone the whole merits of the Turkish Bath may be safely based. Its partisans need seek no other. Herein alone rests its all-sufficient defense.

Some of the facts on which the true philosophy of the Turkish Bath is based may be easily comprehended, and very briefly summed up.

The blood, as is well understood, describes a two-fold circuit in the body. 1st, that through the lungs; 2d, that through the general system. The heart, a double organ, and as a great force-pump for each circle, is placed at the junction between the two. But, mark well, the propulsive power or force-pump function of the heart, extends only a comparatively small way in the route the blood has to travel, *i. e.*, only through the more capacious trunks and palpable vessels. When we come to the *capillary circulation* (which is by far the greater moiety of the whole) we find *supplementary local forces* invoked to aid the transit of the vital fluid. We say nothing here of the alleged influence of the ganglionic nerves—of the contractile power of the capillaries—of the affinities and reactions existing between the vessels and their contents. These may be good hypotheses, but they are not demonstrable agents. The grand motor power we have now to introduce, viz., *cutaneous and pulmonary transpiration, is* demonstrable and point blank. There is an exact analogy and

co-relation between the functions of the leaf in plants
and those of the skin and lungs of animals. [The lungs
may be likened to an extended inward skin, rolled up
into folds or convolutions, *honeycomb-wise*, for the purpose of close packing]

Now, the force or influence which promotes the as-
cent of the sap in plants—viz., the exhalation from the
the leaf—is one identical physical principle with that
which determines the motion of the fluids of the body
toward the exterior, viz., the transpiration from the
skin and lungs. All liquids in connection with an
evaporating membrane acquire motion towards that
membrane. In other words, evaporation from living
surfaces, or even from dead membranes in contact with
liquids, causes the fluids to rise in the capillaries, thus
producing motion or determination from behind, *i. e.*,
from within toward the surface. The amount of motion is directly proportionate to the rapidity of evaporation, *i. e.*, stands in a fixed relation to the temperature
and moisture, or dryness of the atmosphere. Capillary
attraction fills the vessels, but it does not cause the
fluids to rise. The motion of the fluids belongs to, or
is derived from, the evaporating surface. The immense
transpiration constantly going on, in the state of health,
from the large exhalant surface of the skin and lungs,
produces a virtual vacuum within the capillary tubes
whence the fluid or vapor is oozing. By the external
pressure of the atmosphere, and in the case of the
lungs, by the vacuum created at each expiration, the
fluids are forced, or rather drawn, into the superficial
vessels. In this way the blood acquires a decided
movement and determination to the surface. This *vis
ab extra* is no doubt aided by the other powers con

cerned in the circulation, as the contraction of the capillaries, the chemico-vital actions taking place in their extremities, &c., &c.

From all this it will be very apparent how the suppression of transpiration (as by improper exposure to chills and draughts when the skin is unfortified or bathed in sweat, or by states of the atmosphere in which moisture and heat or cold coincide; and, therefore, the conditions of evaporation fail) is followed, as a necessary consequence, by a check of this outward movement of the fluids. A primary essential of health, if not of life, is thus interfered with. If the power of vital resistance be not strong, or if, at the same time, the body be diseased and weakened, then occurs sanguineous arrest or stagnation—congestions of vital organs, and, in the same proportion, impairment of vital functions. The lay-reader will not marvel at the fatality of lung diseases, chronic or acute, when he reflects that the lungs are a great rolled-up inner skin,* with tubes, like the branches and twigs of a tree, penetrating in all directions through that rolled-up mass— a true congeries of cells to convey the air to its hidden surfaces and convolutions. Bronchitis coats over the lining of this branching air-tube with a viscid phlegm. Pneumonia solidifies the porous mass of cells which constitutes, as it were, the leaves of this imaginary tree. Apoplexy floods this whole structure with blood. Tubercle compacts and hardens the mass. It is a con-

---

*Imagine a great net of the finest texture and material, some fifty yards of blood, for example, with a minute but very distinct bladder filling up each mesh, and all this rolled up into the size and shape of a sugar loaf; but from the apex or cone (the point) proceeds a tube, with dividing branches and twigs, precisely like those of a tree, penetrating the congeries of cells and blood vessels in all directions, to convey the air to its every convolution, and to its inmost recesses. This gives you a perfect idea, if a rough one, of the lungs.

cretion in its effect equivalent to sealing up or obstructing the pores of the skin *with a close crop of warts.* In
such a state of affairs how can transpiration take place?
What becomes of the functions of the lungs thus beset?
Imagine a large patch of these supposed warts, ulcerat-
ing and bleeding, and coalescing into a seething crater
of corruption, and the general disturbance and local
desolation that will emanate from this morbid centre
There you have the essence of consumption—what may
be called, after this figure of speech, the Ætna or
Vesuvius of the living man, rather say of the dying
man! Even, without a figure, we talk of pulmonary
caverns.

No fact, then, we think, can be established more
clearly than this, viz., that whatever impedes exhalation from the cutaneous surface, or from the air-cells
of the lungs, stagnates the circulation of the blood
in the interior organs. If the stoppage of the exhalation be complete, the arrest of the circulation is
entire and sudden. Death, with coldness and shivering, ensues. Hence we find that coating over a rabbit
with pitch (by preventing exhalation, and, therefore,
the circulation and oxygenation of the blood) rapidly
diminishes its heat, in fact, asphyxiates it. The rabbit
so treated dies in a shivering fit!

We have another beautiful illustration of this doctrine of suppressed transpiration in the phenomena of
epidemic cholera. Whatever be the noxious agent or
miasm that causes the disease, one thing is very certain, viz., that it operates to annul or paralyze at once
both pulmonary and cutaneous exhalation. Hence, the
Turkish Bath, early had recourse to, would be the cure

par excellence, as it cuts short the cold stage of ague.
The stifling old fashioned vapor and hot-air baths,
under the bed-clothes, failed because what was wanted
was pure hot oxygen, and the lungs to have their due
share of it. The essential of cholera is the draining
away of the watery portion of the blood by the exhalant surface of the bowels! What remains is so much
clot, or tar-like residuum that cannot circulate. The
lungs are useless and the skin dead. Transpiration is
abolished. Oxygenation is impossible. The living
furnace won't draw! The carbon cannot be burnt off.
Animal heat cannot be elaborated. Hence the deathly
coldness and blue skin characterizing the disease, from
the entirely venous nature of the contents of the
vessels. When things have come to this pass the
vitality of the blood is reduced to the lowest ebb.
Hence the simple chemical affinities gain the ascendant
over the vital. The serum of the blood separates from
the fibrine, and the channel of its outlet once being
opened from the congested intestinal membrane (where
the blood has retreated on being driven from the surface) there is nothing in the unaided powers of the
constitution to stop the drain of vitality. The salts of
the serum indeed *operate as a cathartic* to each exhalant tube! The drain goes on so long as there is any
serum to drain away. The primary conditions of life
fail, the organic powers are brought to a stand. The
system sinks, defeated in an unequal contest.*

*Yet even in this, the body's direst extremity, if the patient has not been
already poisoned by the remedies, or if the constitution has not been impaired
by excesses, or by chronic visceral irritation (as from drugging and dram-
drinking), genial nature will usually come to the rescue. The vomiting and
purging will stop from sheer exhaustion, from there being no more serum to
drain away. The very collapse that follows gives the organism time to rally —
to collect her forces for a final struggle with the enemy. In the calm that

But the evil of checked transpiration does not lie solely in the visceral congestions so produced; but there is, moreover, the arrest of the chemico-vital changes ever operating, both on the surface and in the interior of the body. Perspiration, for example, contains, as we have already remarked, lactic acid and the lactates of soda and ammonia—the products of the decay of the muscular tissues in which this acid abounds. During muscular exertion these products are largely evolved. Hence, if perspiration be checked under such circumstances, by prolonged cold, or chill, then these decomposed materials are retained in the blood, or forced to be eliminated by the vicarious duty of other organs. This is the fountain and origin of

---

follows, the soft tissues constituting the greater part of the body, yield up the fluids that yet saturate them, and the salutary thirst created brings fresh supplies. The vessels receive the new tribute, and contract down upon their diminished contents, and so the circulation once more recommences. The reaction is apt to be excessive—a grand source of peril in the convalescence.

We cannot dismiss this allusion to the cholera question without bearing an honest but fearless and emphatic testimony to the merits of Dr. William Stevens, the discoverer of the only true antidote yet found to the ravages of this fearful scourge of mankind. His *saline treatment* constitutes one of the finest illustrations of the application of the Baconian or inductive method of philosophy, to disease and remedy, to be found in the whole range of medical science. In fact, the medication in question is, perhaps, the only instance of a *specific* in the practice of the Art of Physic furnished. Everywhere else we grope more or less in the dark as to the real *modus operandi* of medicines. But here, the precise ingredients that are drained away in the exuded serum of the blood are restored to .t! The success of the treatment corresponds with the accuracy of the philosophical analysis that dictated it—only two or three per cent. of failures—while a host of rival modes of cure often lose one-half of the cases; sometimes three-fourths! But impartial historical truth compels us to confess that paltry professional jealousy and personal pique were long permitted to obscure this great discovery, and to rob the suffering public, to a great extent, of its benefits. In this he only resembles his great prototypes, Harvey and Jenner. Posterity will do him justice. Advanced now "in age and feebleness extreme"—his heart dead and his ear deaf to the voice of human applause, he may yet console himself that a grateful country will not quite let his memory die! It would have been, perhaps, sufficient for the glory of a lesser name, to have been among the first—if not the very first—of surgeons who planned and successfully executed the grand operation of *tying the internal iliac artery!*

rheumatism, gout, diseases of the kidneys and skin, erysipelas, fevers, inflammations, etc. Hence we see how the blood becomes doubly tainted, doubly charged with abnormal elements. The oppressed excretory organs are far from being up to the mark of their own respective functions, let alone performing supernumerary duty. Digestion and assimilation are weakened in the same proportion. Herein is a new and independent source of the direct generation of morbid products. Thus is the *melee* of the suffering organism thickened, and confusion gets worse confounded.

3d. *The Liver.* As this is a great decarbonizing organ, supplementary to the skin and lungs, and one influenced powerfully by the Turkish Bath, its function falls necessarily for review in this place. Situated midway between the apparatus of supply and the organs of distribution, it acts as a reservoir of carbon and a *diverticulum* from the heart and lungs, straining off, before it reaches these organs, the surplusage of carbon brought by the *mesenteric veins* directly from the alimentary canal. But the liver does something more than rid the system, at first hand, of superfluous carbon. The bile is more than an excrementitious fluid. Before being ejected, it is turned to account for the purpose of digestion. Thus is the liver wisely ordained to economize material, to subserve nutrition, even by refuse drainage matter. It serves to sift and clarify the dissolved contents of the stomach and bowels. It checks the influx, into the general system of excess of carbon coming directly from the sources of supply, and so takes the strain off of organs already sufficiently charged with the body's impurities. The *thoracic duct*, or great main-pipe of the lacteal system, carries the chyle (the newly absorbed nutrient principles) directly to the venous trunk terminating in the heart. But the otherwise disposable carbon is absorbed by the mesenteric veins, and so finds summary exit by the liver—multitudinous and complex ends accomplished by simple means that show wondrous design—mingled Wisdom and Goodness. The immense quantity of blood the liver receives from the coats of the intestines, and which it decarbonizes, places in a strong light the relief the due performance of its allotted work affords to its coadjutors, the skin and lungs. These three grand allies in the living economy intimately co-operate with each other, play into each other, substitute each other, sympathize with each other, suffer with each other, and have their diseases cured by the relief of each other. The failure of any one of this "triple alliance" imposes upon the other's vicarious duty, *i. e.*, if they can do it; and where they cannot, disease is the consequence. The prevalence of liver complaints among the indolent, luxurious, and high-fed classes, and in Europeans living in hot climates after the dietetic fashion of cold countries, is not now difficult to account for. In the first place, their food abounds in rich carbonaceous compounds, the error being not less in quantity than quality. In the second place, the amount of stimulent liquors taken to propel along their heavy indigestible meals, aggravates the intestinal irritation by determining an undue amount of blood in the alimentary mucous membrane. In this case, the skin loses what the intestine gains; the sanguineous excess of the one causing its deficit in the other. In the third

place the want of adequate exercise of the limbs, lungs
and skin, fills up the measure of these evils. This it
does by preventing that due waste of the body, that
activity of the excernant functions which passes off
with the least bane to the constitution, the superfluities
of a full or pernicious diet, oxydizing and eliminating
the impededed products of decomposition. Herein
precisely lies the error people commit in hot weather
at home, or in burning climates abroad. Herein is
the philosophy of the bilious diseases then and there
prevalent. Under a high temperature the cutaneous
functions require the most unimpeded scope, instead
of being diminished or paralyzed by diversions of
blood to the interior by congested mucous membranes,
etc., all the effects of table excesses, of irritant food,
drinks or drugs. Hence the two-fold source of the
accumulation of carbon in the system. 1st, that in
the liver directly, from a too heating, full and fatty
diet, especially in warm weather or in hot climates.
2nd, that in the general circulation, or in congested
viscera, from its impeded exit by the skin and lungs.
In cold weather, on the other hand, or in cold climates,
people are less bilious. The habits are necessarily
much more active, to enable them to resist the cold.
The limbs, lungs and skin are all in more vigorous
play, and so effecting more completely corporeal waste,
as well as throwing it out, burning up the fuel of the
living furnace, exalting animal heat by quickened
transformation of matter, and the increased chemico-
vital changes so brought about. To this extent, therefore, is the liver relieved of the supplementary duty it
would otherwise be obliged to assume, if the superficial outlets of carbon were locked up or acting under

par. Hence, in cold weather, the comparative, if not complete immunity from bilous disorders of persons of temperate and active habits. But in hot seasons or climates, there being little or no demand for carbonaceous diet as fuel to heat the body, the labor of its extra extrication must necessarily fall chiefly on the liver. Hence, this organ, taken aback by duty it is incompetent for, irritated and overtasked, falls into disorder. Nature often attempts to clear away the surplusage thus accumulated, in the shape of cholera, dysentery, diarrhœa, fevers, etc. The same explanation accounts for the popularity of such medicines as calomel, colchicum, dandelion, etc., that stimulate the functions of the liver and emulge its ducts. These intestinal irritants and disgorgers of loaded gall bladder and bile-tubes, afford the needed relief, but it is only temporary. It is like borrowing cash in the Palmer fashion, at 600 per cent! But say only cent. per cent. interest, or fifty per cent., what follows? What must follow but corporeal bankruptcy sooner or later? The spend-thrift goes on for a time, leaning on the false prop that is to pierce and break him. Medicinal stimulents, like alcoholic, leave behind the necessity for their repetition in increased dose. And, note well, the stomach was never intended to be a depository of filth in any shape, and pharmaceutical filth is often the most abominable of all. The stomach is only fitted, as designed, to receive the legitimate elements of the corporeal structures—the sound building materials of the body. Aught else is inappropriate, unassimilable, uncongenial; in fact, in a lesser or greater degree, acts as a poison, if it be not actually such. This is a principle that cannot be impugned. But this game of over-stimulating, over-helping, over-straining the liver, will not always continue. The day of reckoning comes at last. Long enduring Nature gets into the *sulks*; she will endure and be "put upon" no longer. Functional derangement, under all this tampering and tinkering, ends in structural alteration. A prime organ of life gives way, profound general malaise and disorder follow in its train, and the whole fabric totters to its fall.

The biliary disturbances, whether periodical or continued, is the simple attempt to explode off the pent up materials of disease; and in sooth, what are most diseases but efforts of nature to rid the system of substances undrawn off by the excretories, by the outlets appointed to eliminate whatever is superfluous or injurious? In a state of the system so charged and ready for a morbid explosion, it is easily conceivable how little things may upset the nice balance of health, may drop a spark of fire, as it were, among combustibles; as, for example, an indigestible article of food, a convivial excess, mental worry, extreme heat or cold, etc. It is not so clearly apparent how the same cause, in one case, insinuates slow, lingering but fatal disorder, and in another, carries off the patient by rapid cholera, inflammation, rheumatic, typhoid, .or putrid fever, etc., etc.

A vast deal of low spirits, *ennui, tœdium vitœ*, etc., of the easy and wealthy classes, arises sheerly from the deficient excretion of the body's waste, notably from accumulated carbon, from biliary impurities; the freest, best and safest vent to which would be by the skin, as roused by the Turkish Bath. If these morbid accumulations were sudden, they would produce all the shock of a narcotic poison, sometimes immediate death or paralysis; but, accummulated piecemeal, the system gets time to accommodate itself to the poison, as it does with alcohol, or opium, or arsenic, in large doses, if gradually begun with and long persevered in. But this very tolerance on the part of the constitution is the cause of the digestive and biliary derangements of the over-fed and under-worked classes. With so palpable a _materies morbi_ gorging the liver, floating in the circulation and poisoning its life springs, its particles arrested, perhaps, in the delicate textures of the brain, is it any marvel that patients are consumed with all sorts of nondescript bodily aches and ails—worst of all, with mental misery, far more intolerable than corporeal suffering? "A peerage or a pension," as the _Times_ would say to the physician who should successfully exorcise these demons of our high civilization, the plagues of our most refined society. In the Turkish Bath,* conjoined with diet and regimen, air, exercise, and discipline of the appetites and passions, lies the remedy.

---

* Well regulated, _bien entendue_, and not prescribed at random, or to be invoked at the beck or whim of every patient who has once experienced its solaces. I happen to know that already the bath, like other good things, is being abused. Thus, a good cause will, bye and bye, get discredited.

CHAPTER III.

It is a sound axiom, universally received and acted
upon by philosophical physicians, viz., that the disordered organism, given fair play to, rights itself;
rectifies its own derangements; and it is, therefore, a
principle held by some of the great practitioners of our
time, one ably contended for by the late Sir John
Forbes, that the cure of disease may be legitimately
sought for in the due use of Nature's pure elements
(*i. e.*, in the appointed or physiological stimuli of the
vital powers; in the judicious aiding, abetting and sustentation of those powers in their self-conservative
struggles) and not exclusively in the vain nostrums and
farragos of the apothecary's art! These may be all
good in their place. The alleged " specifics " are non-
entities, are a fallacy, a delusion and a snare! We
have no specifics. Science renounces the research.
Not more nonsensical was the pursuit of the " Elixir
Vitæ," the "Aurum Potabile," the " Philosopher's
Stone." My Lord Palmerston would define to a T the
function of the physician *as being " the judicious bottle-
holder" to Nature.'* This is really, in a great crowd of
cases, the grand part he has to act. Now, we shall
see what salutary ingredients the Turkish Bath puts
into this restorative bottle: how it relieves Nature
of the impediments that shackle her operations, how it

softens and relaxes the solids that the fluids may the more freely circulate, how it expands and opens up the vast porous structure of the tissues, and so promotes the clearance and cleansing of the secret rills, and channels, and reservoirs of life. It sensibly seeks to purify the vital currents by flushing the vital sewers! It opens up the waste-pipes of the body, only to run off and disgorge through them its accumulated filth. The pores of the skin constitute, in fact, the vastest drainage system of the animal economy, and are at once the safest route and most salutary outlet for purging off all extraneous, decomposed, or superfluous matters. The Turkish Bath sets about this scavenger-work by the immersion of the body in pure hot air. A preliminary macerating, sweating, clarifying, and eliminating process is thus performed. The pores are again closed, and the relaxed tissues and skin contracted, tonified and braced up by tepid, then cold ablutions. Renovated vigor is thus imparted to the whole organism, even without the refreshment of food! Thus a grand immediate benefit is gained by this truly artistic process, viz., to nourish and strengthen the body upon the old materials existing in the storehouses of the fabric, to burn them off, or to use them up, so as in any case to have clear receptacles and clear conduits for the elaboration and distribution of the new food. In this way we notably energize or activate the absorbing powers, the threefold effect of which is: first, to promote perfect circulation; second, to break up and remove unhealthy tissues; and third, to put down more substantial structures in their place.

It may be received as a companion proposition to the first we stated under the present head of our subject—

perhaps almost as a corollary from it, viz , that all
irritation by drugs, violent corrosive substances (or by
concentrated alcoholic stimulants), of the delicate internal lining of the alimentary canal is equivalent to
blistering it ! Give a strong healthy dog a dose of
what is considered a " mild domestic" medicine—
" grey powder," with castor oil, or salts and senna.
Dissected the day after, the mucous membrane of the
intestines will present, here and there, large blood-shod
patches—telling how the blister has acted. And yet
we every day so blister the gastric tubes of delicate
infants and children—not to talk of the horse-blister-
ing in the case of adults—by aloes and colocynth,
calomel and drastic salts, scammony and gamboge,
elaterium and tartar emetic, Croton oil, *et hoc genus
omne*.

Now, the Turkish Bath is wholly antagonistic to this
destructive stimulation of the most delicate, sensitive,
and highly vitalized surfaces of the body ; tissues
" tender as the apple of the eye"—as repellant to rude
touch—as resentful of abrasion—and as difficult to
appease when irritated. But the Bath not only does
not irritate, it positively soothes man's sentient inner
and outer linings, at the very time that it opens, and
flushes and floods the body's natural drains.

As the internal organs, therefore, are nice things to
tamper with, or rather won't safely bear tampering
with, Nature sets before us the skin as the grand battle-
field in the warfare with disease. The keeping of this
field in proper trim is also the best means of preserving
health regained or not yet forfeited. Everywhere else
the system may be refractory to our operations, and

impatient or irresponsive to discipline; but the skin is always placable, always submissive, ever ready to be soothed or coaxed; and failing that, is not unwilling to be coerced into salutary action for the rest of the economy; provided, always we know the right way to evoke its powers and to conciliate its co-operation.

The most fertile sources of morbid elements in the blood are retained or altered secretions. These are now admitted to lie at the foundation of a great majority of diseases; hence, the most theoretically-feasible as well as the most practically-available agents of cure are those required for the healthy exercise of the natural functions, especially those of waste and repair—of secretion and excretion. In the capillaries chiefly, if not exclusively, are carried on these processes of waste and repair—the building up of the new fabrics, and the taking down and taking away of the old, worn-out, or useless materials of the body. Now the principal, —at least the most demonstrable—seat of action of the Turkish Bath, is the capillary system; its grand effect is thoroughly to open and cleanse the capillary tubes and strainers—to clear out their obstructions, and freely to circulate the blood through them.

The chief help Nature requires in most diseases, chronic and acute, is first, to open the safety-valves, to rid the body of its impurities; then to establish the equilibrium of the blood alike in the central and superficial parts of the body—to sooth the sentient external surface, and to allay internal irritation—to relieve laboring viscera of intropelled fluids (*i. e.*, of congestion or stagnation.) This purifying process, this inward unloading of organs, this equable distribution

of the blood, is the sure, if not necessary, result
of active determination to the exhalant surfaces, and
the powerful drain therefrom of fluids easily and
promptly replaceable.

Now, these aims just specified are the the curative
aims and "indications" of all medical practice, no
matter what outward badge the practitioner may wear
—what sect he follows—what name he is called by.
That which best accomplishes these aims must needs
be the best curative agent. The Turkish Bath, we
conceive, unquestionably makes good this pretension,
and is, therefore, the agent that comes nearest to the
beau ideal of curative art. Above all other systems of
healing, it is *par excellence* the equalizer of the circulation—the unrivalled and unfailing derivative to the
surface—the solvent of capillary engorgements—the
dissipator of morbid accumulations—the opener up of
the body's safety-valves, and the flusher of its common sewers and drains ; in short, the clean sweeper-out
of all filth blocking up the life-channels and poisoning
the life-springs.

These are the direct and immediate effects of the
practice we advocate. The indirect and the remote
effects are, the increased quantity and improved
quality of the secretions, the regulation of nutrition,
and, in a word, the exaltation of vitality in the whole
organism. In this way alone, can we rationally hope
so to aid and sustain nature as that she will be able
to throw off most of the diseases that assail the fabric.

How, then, does the Turkish Bath accomplish all
these salutary effects? How does it establish claims
to efficacy such as no drugs and no system of medicine

can pretend to? All this we shall proceed now to explain.

The first essential element of the action of the Turkish Bath is hot air; the purer the atmospheric oxygen, and the freer of all admixture or dilution, clearly the better. Under this stimulus, the whole secretory activity of the system is roused, transpiration is powerfully increased, both from the skin and lungs, with the effect of imparting extra activity to the circulation —a point sufficiently established in describing the effects of exhalation from the surface of the leaf in plants. This sanguineous *molimen*, or determination, is not merely on the surface; but it is effected from within, and to the surface. Every vital, vegetative, or purely organic function is stirred up to unwonted activity; the heart beats with renewed energy, and the blood vessels participate in its augmented impulse. The skin at length opens apace, however bound, obstructed, or reluctant its outlets at first may have been. With the pouring forth of perspiration, and thereby the absorption or neutralization of an immense amount of the surplus or latent heat of the body, comes instantaneous relief—a subsidence of the whole physiological tumult, raised expressly, as it were, to drive out an intruder. The large demand for vital fluids set up on the surface, and the chemico-vital elaborations there taking place, tend powerfully to unlock and draw away the pent up blood of diseased interior structures, congested viscera, and the like. The "change of matter," or "the transformation of the tissues"' over the whole body is facilitated; in other words, the waste of the animal structures is largely augmented. This demands the quicker elimination of this waste. With the increased outpouring of the structural debris,—veritable body sewage—unhealthy elements imprisoned within are loosened, set afloat, and swept off by this real flood-tide of fluids,* speeding onward to the surface, like rivers, to be lost and exhaled in the ocean. The completeness of the aeration of the blood corresponds in degree to the activity of exhalation; respiration is deepened, and the lungs are profoundly filled.† These actions now described are the most powerfully alterative we know. The effect on nutrition, the correction of its aberrations, is not long to manifest itself.

All this profuse drain of liquids oozing out by every pore of the surface, and drawn from every depth and cranny of the interior, justifies and calls for proportionate supplies of water by way of drink. This new fluid in its turn is drained away—thus literally washing out the blood, dissolving and straining off its impurities, and scouring out even the vessels. Absorbtion, therefore, is not less quickened than elimination. Renewal and waste thus run a race with recruited powers. No morbid humors, or even hard deposits, can long stand this perturbative, or break up process, pro-

---

* *Suspended internal functions* of various sorts have thus a *chance* of being set free from fetters that may have long enthralled them; and with this vent given to pent-up nature, the bloom of youth is restored to many a pallid cheek, especially in the case of young females. The simple draining-off of the overabundant watery elements of the blood of the subjects in question is no mean service rendered to the constitution, and paves the way for the filling of the vessels with purer and healthier materials. Of course, to do these cases full justice, they should be under professional superintendence.

† Hence the beneficial effects that may be legitimately expected in chronic congestion, hepatization, tubercular deposits, etc., of the pulmonary organs. But as these are the nicest of all cases to treat, they require careful surveillance, as well as accurate diagnosis. No random dosing will do; otherwise debility, rather than strength, may soon result.

vided only it be judiciously repeated, so as not to impair the strength, or exhaust the stamina of the subject. In this way excessive fatty deposition is broken up, melted down, and swilled out of the system, gross morbid humors of various kinds, and unhealthy tissues, are absorbed and removed. The muscles are rendered more compact; the skin tenser, more elastic, more clear, more glossy, more satiny, as well as more permeable. The same activity of absorption which takes down the paunchy and the bloated, also promotes the fattening of the lean and ill-nourished. and this, not only because the nutrient materials in the stomach are turned to better account, but because their resorption into the circulation is more energetic.

We have made no reference here to the action of the Turkish Bath on the Great Sympathetic System of Nerves. The stimulus of heat must powerfully affect these nerves, as well as the ganglionic and common sensory nerves. In like manner acts the stimulus of cold, which is also an integral and essential part of the Bath. The organic functions, or the purely vital and vegetative actions of the economy, are much under the influence of the grand sympathetic and ganglionic nerves; and, therefore, it is to be inferred that we could have no increase of circulation, exhalation, secretion, etc, without the stimulation of these nerves. It may be demonstrated another day that in this sympathetic and ganglionic stimulation lies the whole curative virtue of the Turkish Bath, inasmuch as it is the forerunner and exciting cause of the augmented physiological actions that constitute the peculiar phenomena of the Bath.

The shampooing process, if not an essential, is a

usual accompaniment of the Turkish Bath. Skilfully and moderately performed, as befits the less pliable frames of the hardier nations of the West, it will necessarily receive due attention, especially wherever the grand object of the Bath is to substitute exercise. But the subject simply requires allusion to here, not elucidation. At the end of the above described macerating ordeal—when the muscles, blood-vessels, nerves and skin are all relaxed—is the proper time for kneading the body, in the same way as iron is best moulded and welded, and fashioned, when hot—an apt simile of Mr. Urquhart's.

The bracing, fortifying discipline of tepid and cold ablutions properly succeeds to the preliminary procedure of stirring up the circulating system, softening the surface, opening the pores, and producing purgation and waste by the skin. After thus giving vent to effete matters, or retained excretions, this conclusion of the process and closure of the pores, is a *sine qua non* of the Turkish Bath—following up and confirming its benefits. Without this finale, its efficacy would be impaired, if not forfeited or lost, for a great many subjects. The unreflecting, or the totally inexperienced, may shrink at the idea of this sudden transition from high temperature to a cold bath, as something dreadful to bear or dangerous to practice. But it is neither the one nor the other. The fear is a fallacy; the apprehension entirely groundless. On the contrary the application of cold, after perspiration in this fashion (passive) is not only not dangerous, but it is highly salutary and refreshing—exhilarating, in truth, beyond any previous conception of the uninitiated.

This conclusive operation is based on the soundest physiology, and is not less needful and appropriate than it is grateful to the patient. A general maceration of the tissues has been effected. The vessels, and nerves, and skin, have been all relaxed from the heat and stimulation they have been subjected to, and from the copious floods that have oozed through them. A virtual depletion has been effected, the only depletion that is sound and safe. Now, then, is demanded, and is borne, the shock—the bracing power of cold. By this the cerebro-spinal and ganglionic nerves have temporary excess of vitality at once imparted to them—a veritable electric thrill is felt. A rush of blood is determined to the surface, to replace the heat abstracted. The effect of this is to increase and fix the circulation in the skin, thus rousing the capillary actions of the surface at the expense of the interior; promoting thereby the dispersal of congestions, and establishing the sanguineous equilibrium of the central and superficial parts of the body. All this brings about a rapid "transformation of the tissues," the breaking up, absorption, and swilling out of old, decayed or diseased matters, and the deposition of new. The normal, or physiological activity of the vital functions is increased—the *vis vitæ* exalted everywhere. The more freely the skin has been acting, the larger the flow of fluids, the greater will be the cold that is desired; the better will it be borne; the more potent will be the stimulus it affords; the more permanent the re-action that will ensue; the more decided, in short, its curative results. Hence the feeling of immense relief and solace, of renovated mental

and corporeal vigor, after a process that, to the superficial thinker, seems exhausting.

The phenomena above described are vaguely expressed by the word reaction. In this reaction itself
lies a great aim and agency of cure. To be able
to react well is the grand help nature requires in a
majority of diseases. The body corporeal then does
for itself, for its enemies within, what the body politic
does for itself when it rises *en masse* to repel its
enemies without. In both cases, the effect is at least
to quell or appease internal irritations, dissensions and
tumults !

By the discipline of the Bath, any over-sensitiveness
or morbid sensibility of the skin becomes so blunted,
its tissues are so braced and fortified, its natural
functions so exalted, as to bear with impunity any
transitions of temperature, and the more extreme,
often the more agreeable ; as also the more hardening
the effect. With the restoration of a high condition
of the skin, coincides the return of healthy functions
in the mucous linings, whether of the lungs or of the
alimentary canal. In this way persons that are subject, on slight exposure, to catarrh, influenza, bronchitis, diarrhœa, etc., get case-hardened to atmospheric
variations, and even bear draughts with impunity.

The allegation that perspiration is a weakening process is another fallacy that hardly needs demolition.
Sweating, as accomplished by drugs (sudorifics), we
admit, is a debilitating drain. So is the vapor bath as
used in the bungling way common in our old bath
establishments. But properly evoked, and followed
by tepid and then cold ablutions, it is, on the contrary,

highly tonic and invigorating. In the Turkish Bath, the patient lies full-stretched, in perfect repose, on couch, bench, or *dureta*. Nothing of the normal constituents of the body is abstracted save the saline and watery portions of the blood. The water is replaced by absorption from the stomach as rapidly as it is given out; for, when the drain comes to be excessive, the supply is proportionate. And here, be it well observed, it is only in very pure systems that the water, welling out from the pores, comes away pure. It is far otherwise when the body is impure. Not only the water oozed out by the pores, but the atmosphere all around is tainted by the eliminated products and exhalations of disease. This happens in bad cases of chronic maladies, characterized by corrupt humors, constitutional taints, etc., *i. e.*, whenever the secreting and excreting functions are materially interfered with; whenever, in short, substances are retained either in the highways or the byways of the circulation that should have been eliminated. These constitute a very formidable, as a very palpable and intelligible *materies morbi*. In granular kidney (Bright's Disease) these odors in the calidarium are occasionally something dreadful. The easy exit afforded to these pent-up elements of disease by the powerful drains and perturbative action of the Turkish Bath is, beyond all contradiction, the source of its immediate and permanent benefits. Hence, if skilfully wielded, the reputation it is likely to achieve in the cure of visceral congestions, morbid accumulations and obstructions, and in blood-taints, etc.

If the Bath fails, nothing else will avail to transfer to the robbed, emptied, shrivelled, parchment-like

surface of the body, blood long pent-up in a torpid
liver, an engorged spleen, a congested mucous membrane, or a hepatized lung. By its outlet of peccant
matters it gives immediate relief to *malaise*, misery
and fatigue. Increased absorption and elimination
remarkably improve the appetite, and promote digestion and nutrition; healthier solids and fluids are
formed than those that are thrown out or wasted
down. Hence, the Turkish Bath fills up the skinny or
flabby, and reduces the obese, the paunchy, and the
plethoric.

THE LEGITIMATE MEDICAL DOMAIN OF THE TURKISH BATH—ITS PRACTICAL APPLICATIONS.

The Turkish Bath is the truest and best anti-spas-
modic. In cramps of all degrees; in spasms of the
muscles of the bowels, which are the source of the
pains called colic; in spasms of the gall-bladder and
gall-ducts; in pains in the region of the kidneys, or
lumbago; in spasms of the bronchial tubes (asthma);
even in lock-jaw and tetanus, its use is a legitimate
and hopeful experiment at least. Between the combined effects of the hot room and cold douche, spasms
of any sort will have a better chance of yielding than
under any other mode of treatment; but very hot
fomentations with flannel must be conjoined. In any
case, the tedious convalescence, the usual result of the
powerful medicines swallowed to overcome spasms,
will be saved.

The Bath presents a valuable resource in the reduction of dislocations, and of strangulated hernial tumors
(ruptures).

The Bath will be of the greatest utility in passive diseased states, wherever action is below par, as in the very commencement of accute diseases, in the premonitory stage of fevers and inflammations—the stage of depression of power—in the congestive stages of eruptive diseases (measles, scarlet fever, small pox, etc.,) wherever, in short, collapse takes place and the symptoms show retrocession of the fluids from the surface to the interior; in other words, wherever congestion of vital organs exists or is apprehended.

The Turkish Bath, for this reason, is an unquestionable resource in cholera—will be, perhaps, its grand remedy in the first stage. Having already spoken at large of this disease, as likely to be influenced by the Turkish Bath, we need not enlarge here.

The Turkish Bath should be at once had recourse to in the collapse, shivering uneasy feelings and depressed spirits that follow a decided chill of the surface, when perspiring freely; as, for example, when getting wet in an exhausting journey, or from the absorption into the lungs of an infectious miasm—a dose of which a man often gets in standing over an open drain. In all these cases, before active irritation or acute inflammatory symptoms have manifested themselves, there is every reason to hope that many diseases would be strangled (to use the favorite phrase of French practitioners) at the very off-go, and thus many premature deaths, often of the most illustrious personages, would be prevented. Thus died the Duke of Kent! Thus died George Washington! Thus died Count Mirabeau! and thousands of others.

In purely nervous irritations of the heart, or in

those connected with organic disease, in simple palpitations; in *angina pectoris*, the hot room actually does quiet the circulation, and would do so still more remarkably, we think, if the cold or hot compress, according to circumstances, were kept on the chest and often refreshed.

In the case of local spasms, hot flannel fomentations applied to the seats of suffering while in the tepidarium would probably facilitate their solution.

The Turkish bath will diminish the liability to take infectious diseases. This often depends upon a habitually sluggish condition of the kidneys, with marked and scant secretion. The powerful revulsion to the surface and drain of fluids by the skin, operated by the Bath, effectually takes the strain off the kidneys— disgorging them, and, in fact, almost performing their functions!

In "Bright's Disease," in diabetes, in gout and rheumatism, and in all kidney diseases, with excess of uric acid and its salts, the practice that carries off the corporeal debris by the skin—and not by irritant drugs acting on the kidneys or the bowels—is the true art and science of their cure. In such cases water-drinking during the bath is strenuously to be insisted upon, inasmuch as the excess of water washes out a corresponding proportion of solid constituents. Thus colchicum, or acetate or nitrate of potash, may be superseded.

In Ague, the Turkish Bath offers the most feasible remedy, as being a disease resulting from diminished secretion of the solids strained off by the kidneys. The probability is, therefore, that a highly active state of the cutaneous functions would eliminate these solid matters of the urine through the surface, even as we find an eczematous eruption occasionally frosted over with crystals of urate of soda.

In tic-doloureux, or neuralgia, the Bath promises great things.

Skin diseases will most probably be removed by a very summary process in the Bath, according to all experience hitherto.   ,

In irritative congestions of the wind-pipe, from public speaking ("preachers' throat," so-called,) the Turkish Bath can hardly fail to be pre-eminently successful; for this disease is usually only symptomatic of a morbid condition of the skin and digestive organs.

In acute affections of the throat and tonsils, even in croup and diphtheria, the Bath will almost invariably save life.

In consumption, the Turkish Bath, fairly tested, will, on the clearest abstract grounds, as well as on the showing of facts, produce the greatest ratio of arrests of the disease. The noxious acids of the alimentary canal are thereby drained out of the system, the air-cells of the lungs are dilated, pulmonary secretions are dried up, internal congestions are dissolved and dissipated, the relaxed skin braced, appetite promoted, night perspirations checked, the noxious chills and shivering at once cut short, and refreshing sleep procured.

In digestive derangements characterized by intense acidity, the Turkish Bath offers a great resource, as oozing out through the skin the excess of lactic acid, which often lies at the root of the evils of dyspepsia.

In chronic bronchitis, and emphysema of the lungs, and in the dry catarrh of the aged, the Turkish Bath is worthy of extensive trial.

In dropsies, both of the shut cavities of the bowels and chest, and the exterior tissues, as well as from diseased kidneys, the Turkish Bath is precisely suited and will work wonders—as taking the tension off the veins—the effusion of water being only a vicarious effort to relieve the plethora of the congested vessels.

In tympanitis and other cases of abnormal secretion of gas in the stomach and intestines, the Bath will promote the extrication of the gaseous exhalation, or suppress directly its formation.

In chronic liver disease, in enlargement of the liver, and jaundice, etc., the Turkish Bath will be found the most potent agent of cure, as demonstrated by the large success of the much inferior hydropathic instruments of sweating used in such cases.

In gout and rheumatism the Bath will prove itself the speediest and best remedy.

In syphilis and mercurial diseases ; in diseases arising from the abuse of treatment, the same hydropathic experience calls for an extensive use of the Turkish Bath. The medicated vapor baths of the *Hopital de Midi*, in Paris, are less efficient attempts in the direction of the Turkish Bath.

In the large and too common and distressing class of uterine diseases, the Turkish Bath will supersede, to a very large extent, the often very tedious and (to the constitution) expensive medication, by means of caustic and the knife, mechanical helps, etc.

Cancer has now, perhaps, found its antidote in the Turkish Bath. Mr. Urquhart communicates a remarkable case of a lady who came to him in a desperate and hopeless condition, after the cancer had once been excised, and who was so far recovered as to be able to walk five miles. We hope the profession will give a fair trial to this remedy in a disease wherein they admit the powerlessness of all ordinary agency.

The Turkish Bath will take down, summarily and safely, excessive obesity, literally melting down and oozing out the oil of over-abundant adipose tissues ; draining, as it were, the muscular fibres of this paralyzing accompaniment, as well as thereby increasing the tone and motor-power of these fibres. The Bath promotes the nutrition of the ill-nourished, increasing the appetite in proportion as it increases absorbtion.

In diarrhœa, dysentery, etc., the Bath will be the cure *par excellence;* as determining excessive action and diversion of the fluids from the intestinal lining to the skin, as well as soothing ganglionic irritation.

We are inclined to hope that the Turkish Bath will prove itself the nearest thing to a specific for hydrophobia. If anything will ooze out or neutralize the virus, once perfectly developed, it will be the action of the highest temperature that can be borne. Last century it was the custom, in some parts of Scotland, to smother these unhappy victims, by placing one feather bed upon another, the patient between, and a party of women sitting all around on the edges of the bed. On one of these occasions, within the memory of a living individual, a little boy was put in to be so strangled. After a quarter of an hour, when they thought he was dead, to the surprise of the operators, in taking off the upper bed, he leaped up out of a pool of perspiration in the center of the bed, where he lay, and said he felt quite well—indeed he was cured! This is an encouraging fact for the trial of the Turkish Bath.

The Turkish Bath will undoubtedly prove itself the best corrector of what has been designated the civic cachexia, the vitiated habit of body bred by hard town life, whether it be the life of luxury or the life of labor—a nameless, nondescript condition of the solids and fluids, impairing much, if not quite the relish of life, rendering vapid its enjoyments; and all this the result of over-excited brain, over-worked stomach, over-gorged vessels, and under-worked limbs, lungs and skin—the effect, in a word, of closed safety-valves.

The Turkish Bath will become an indispensable substitute for exercise to three large classes of people: 1st, the indolent and luxurious, who take advantage of their privilege, but who find it, alas! anything but a blessing to be exempt from the primal curse; 2nd, to the brain-toiling, city-pent masses, the keepers at home, the men of literature and science, the drudges of the desk, the prisoners of the counter, or the slaves of the factory; 3d, to valetudinarian multitudes, not

ill enough to be loosened from the cares of business—
" which thousands, once chained to, quit no more,"—
but too ill for personal comfort, and for the comfort
likewise of those around them ; the hypochondriac, the
bilious, the dyspeptic, the bloated, the unwieldy, the
asthmatic, the lame, and the lazy.

From "Winter and its Dangers."

BY DR. HAMILTON OSGOOD, OF NEW YORK.

I must confess to a prejudice against *indiscriminate* use of the Turkish Bath in winter, especially in the rigorous climate of the northern States, unless one can at once go to bed under the same roof. To take such a bath in cold weather, and immediately after go home through a freezing air, is very hazardous, save in the few exceptions which are admitted by even stringent rule. Under the advice and personal direction of a physician, the Turkish Bath, as I am well aware, has often accomplished a good and desired purpose. My objection chiefly refers to unadvised use of it in winter. While it lasts, it is a luxurious delight; but the condition in which it leaves the bather is what makes it dangerous. Notwithstanding the cold affusion which follows the main bath, the body is left in a state of active perspiration, which lasts so long that the majority have not time to wait for its disappearance. This is what makes the bath questionable in winter. I have no objection to offer to it when taken in summer, if due care be exercised and the bather be strong enough to bear its exhausting effects. I have known individuals to faint while the bath was in progress. Delicate and plethoric people, likewise those whose lungs or hearts are weak, should never make use of it.

It is true there is a great temptation in it, for its temporary effects are delicious, and it leaves the skin admirably purified. Indeed, during a first experience in a Turkish Bath, one is involuntarily reminded of Sidney Smith's letter from a hot German bath. "They have already scraped enough off me," he wrote, "to make a curate."

But recently, a well-known gentleman of Boston invited a friend to go with him to see how quickly he would rid himself of a cold. "I am perfectly stiffened by this cold," he said. "Nothing but a Turkish Bath will break it up." It was winter season, for it is then the people are induced to use this bath as a remedy. The gentleman took his bath, and for nearly a month was confined to his chamber. This has been my invariable experience when I have tried to leave a cold in a Turkish Bath. The cold was always worse; and I would earnestly impress upon my readers the danger of this form of bath in winter, unless it be used in a mild climate, or under the eye of a physician.

OUR REPLY.

Some very intelligent physicians could not be more ignorant than they are of the real character and claim of the Turkish Bath if they had made the acquirement of that ignorance a solemn professional duty. An illustration of the truth of this remark may be found in a very valuable and admirable little book by Doctor Hamilton Osgood, of New York, from which the above article was taken. This work is one of the series of American Health Primers, and, while it contains much

that is of the utmost value to the seekers after health,
presents some conclusions respecting the effects of the
Turkish Bath which reveal the presence and influence
of a prejudice which is as unphilosophical as it is unprofessional. The author makes that common mistake
into which the *uneducated* are constantly entrapped,
of believing that two facts stand necessarily in the
relation of cause and effect, when they may exist coin-
cidentally. A shower of rain may follow a fervent
prayer, but it is by no means clear that these two facts
sustain to each other the relation of cause and effect.
In truth, it is becoming plain to an increasingly large
number of thoughtful men that they do not sustain
such a relation. The savage attempts, with noise and
smoke, to drive away the demon which is devouring
the sun during an eclipse, and it is perfectly clear to
the savage that he has succeeded in his benevolent
object, when the great orb emerges from his obscurity
unharmed. But no civilized man shares this conviction. The habit of mind to which I have referred
(and which is so viciously illogical) has done more than
any one single cause to nourish superstition. Thirteen
people sit down to dinner; one of the company dies
before the year is closed. Ergo, Providence objects
to a party of thirteen! A ship leaves port on Friday,
and fails to reach its destination. It is perfectly clear
that voyage should not be begun on that day. We
all remember the sensible reply made by Hotspur to
haughty Glendower The proud Welshman asserts
that he is no common man, because nature was con-
vulsed at his birth. Percy responds, with the declaration, that these natural convulsions would have occurred
if only his *mother's cat had kittened.* Now, the

pertinency of all this will appear when we read Dr. Osgood's wise conclusions touching the Turkish Bath. He says: "I have known individuals to faint while the bath was in progress." So have we. We have known individuals to faint while in church! Comment: Men go to church, because there is something in the character of things social almost certain to produce dizziness and faintness! This is, really, as logical as the Doctor's conclusion. Can the author show, or has it been shown, that the effect described and the cause assigned bear any necessary relationship? Why should a man faint in the Bath? In well-constructed baths the ventilation is perfect and the blood receives its due amount of oxygen. Men are affected injuriously by heat—as in the case of sun-stroke—only when the process of healthy perspiration has been arrested. If a man goes into the bath with a stomach engorged with undigested food, under a state of great nervous excitement, he *may* faint in the bath. So, a man may be violently attacked with nauseau who eats *immoderately* of roast beef and potatoes, but such a result does not impeach the healthfulness and nutritiousness of these articles of food. Nobody claims that one may foolishly violate all these rational and obviously proper conditions under which a bath should be taken, and then justly expect benefit from the remedy. How many of Dr. Osgood's patients would recover if they sought his assistance and advice under the same *intelligent* conditions? It may do no harm to baptize a man in ice-cold water, but if the advice of the old Deacon should be followed and some hardened sinner, newly converted, be "anchored out" over night, he would probably "go to his reward" before morning. Yet, his fate would

present no "awful warning" against the judicious use
of cold water. Dr. Osgood says: "To take such a
bath in cold weather, and immediately after go home
through a freezing air, is very hazardous." We may
add, also, that to get out of a warm bed in your night-
dress and attempt to hold a St. Bernard dog in a snow
bank till he freezes to death, is more hazardous to you
than to the dog! This fact is not generally recognized
by the medical faculty! Why go into the freezing air
immediately? If simply to prove the non-beneficial
effects of the bath, you need not subject yourself to
that inconvenience in order to bring us to conviction.
We have never defended the abuse of the Bath, or the
abuse of any of Heaven's blessings.

Dr. Osgood says: "Under the advice and personal
direction of a physician, the Turkish Bath * * has,
often accomplished a good and desired purpose. My
objection chiefly refers to the unadvised use of it in
winter, * * * * notwithstanding the cold affusion which follows the main bath, the body is left in a
state of active perspiration, which lasts so long that
the majority have not time to wait for its disappearance."

Now the sufficient answer to all this *nonsense*—unpar-
donable in an educated physician—is found in the
presentation of *facts*, not the investigation of theories.
"Why does'nt a two-pound fish increase the weight of a
bucket of water?" asks the scientific theorist. "Well,"
answers Franklin, "let us be sure of the *fact* before
we trouble ourselves with the the theory."

The *facts*—and stubborn ones there are—we have to
present are these: We give from 500 to 700 baths a

month *more in winter* than in summer. The large part of these bathers are *regular* customers, some of them coming as frequently as once a day, though the majority average perhaps twice a week. None of these people (if they have any sense) go "*immediately* into the freezing air," upon leaving the hands of the attendant. But they find, almost invariably, that the "state of active perspiration" does *not* extend beyond thirty minutes, and generally in less than forty-five minutes they are ready to face the "freezing air" with impunity. The "exhausting effects" of the Bath, of which Dr. Osgood speaks, are mainly experienced by those who study the treatment in shallow medical treatises! Why should it exhaust a man to healthfully stimulate the circulation, bring the blood to the surface, and make the skin do part of its work, so frequently crowded upon the kidneys and the liver? We have in our Bath day after day, *in winter*, all kinds and types of people. Fat people, lean people, people with strong lungs, people with weak lungs, fresh and sallow skinned people. They come again and again —have been coming regularly for years, and would never have suspected the deleterious effects of the Bath, had it not been for the *scientific* conclusion of this little book. "Verily," says a grave philosopher, "the only people who know how to bring up children, never have any." So it is plain that the only people who suffer from the "exhausting effects" of the Turkish Baths, *never use them!*

See another brilliant conclusion to which Dr. Osgood has arrived. He says: "A gentleman of Boston had a cold, and he invited a friend to go to the Turkish Bath with him to see how quickly he could cure this cold. This gentleman took his bath. *For nearly a month he was confined to his chamber!*" A sensible person would come to this conclusion: This gentleman had *frequently* cured a cold by the use of the bath, or else he would not have been so confident of its efficacy, and on this occasion *one* bath did *not* avert a months sickness, which circumstances in no way connected with the Bath, had rendered inevitable. We would call Dr. Osgood's attention to the story of the farmer who had eaten four consecutive meals in one day of roast pork, mince pie and toasted cheese, and just before going to bed he consumed four roasted apples. During the night he was brought to the verge of the grave with cramp colic, and the next morning he registered a solemn vow to Heaven, that he would never touch another roasted apple as long as he lived! The doctor may make the application.

THE TURKISH BATH.

This bracing and depurating bath combines many of the properties of the hot and cold bath. The body, subjected to great heat, is made to perspire copiously. If the bath ended here, more or less weakness would ensue; but at this stage the free application of cold water stimulates and braces the body, and produces the tonic effects of the cold bath At each stage of the process, the Turkish Bath cleanses the system; the perspiration carrying off, and the cold consuming, by increased oxydation, many effete and noxious substances in the blood. The baths, says Dr. Goolden, are useful in gout, rheumatism, sciatica, Bright's disease, escema, and psoriasis : they benefit bronchitis, the cough of phthisis, the aching of the muscles from unusual exertion, pains in the seat of old wounds, colds in the head, quinsies, and common winter coughs.

It is not amiss here to caution persons prone to colds, that the habit of over-clothing increases this liability. This cold-catching tendency may be obviated by using a moderate amount of clothing, taking a cold sponge-bath every morning, an occasional wet-sheet packing, or the Turkish Bath once or twice a week.

On catching cold, a patient with lungs previously healthy, becomes troubled for some time with chronic catarrh, accompanied by considerable expectoration and some shortness and oppression of breathing. In such a case, the Turkish Bath generally affords prompt and great relief, checking the expectoration and easing the breathing. In bronchial asthma and emphysematous asthma, a course of Turkish Baths, say one every second or third day, is very useful; this subdues chronic bronchitis and renders the patient less liable to catch cold. A large chamois leather waistcoat reaching low down the body and arms, and worn over the flannel, affords great relief in bronchial asthma and emphysematous bronchitis. This jacket is extremely warm and protects the chest against the vicissitudes of the weather. It is a nasty practice to wear it next the skin.

At the commencement of a feverish cold, a Turkish Bath will cut the attack short, remove the aching pains, and relieve or cure the hoarseness at once. The bath will still prove very useful for a cold of several days' standing, though its good effects are less striking. The Turkish Bath will relieve or carry off the remains of a general severe cold, as hoarseness, cough with expectoration, and lassitude. Whilst in the hot chamber the voice generally becomes quite clear and natural, though the hoarseness may afterwards return in a slight degree; but it usually continues to improve, becoming natural in a day or two, a repetition of the bath aiding complete recovery. In more obstinate cases several baths may be required. Great improvement of the voice in the hot chamber may be taken as proof that the bath will benefit, even though after the bath, the hoarseness returns to a great extent.

The Turkish Bath is serviceable to persons who after dining out, not wisely but too well, suffer next day from *malaise* and slight indigestion. A course of Turkish Baths is very beneficial to towndwellers leading a sedentary life, who, especially if they live freely, are apt to become stout, with soft and flabby tissues, are easily tired, suffer from lack of energy and some mental depression. Under the influence of the bath, their muscles become firmer, the fatness decreases, and they acquire more spirit and energy. A course of Turkish Baths is useful to patients whose health has broken down by residence in a tropical climate, who suffer from general debility, enfeeblement of mind, dull aching pains in the head and broken sleep. I have heard the Turkish Bath, even its daily use, recommended highly for convalescents from acute diseases, to promote assimilation, digestion, and appetite.

Patients suffering from jaundice, acquired in a tropical climate, or from malaria, have often testified to the beneficial effects of Turkish Baths ; but it is necessary as indeed it is with all persons with shattered health, to caution them against the too vigorous and unrestrained use of the bath. The patient should leave the hot chamber as soon as free perspiration occurs, and should not plunge into the cold bath, but take a douche with slightly tepid water, especially in cold weather.

Many dread the Turkish Bath lest they should catch a cold, and one often hears complaints of a cold coming on after a bath. So far from tending to give cold, these baths, as we have said, obviate the tendency to catarrh, and fortify delicate persons with a cold-

catching tendency. If ever the bath is answerable for
a cold, it is almost always owing to the bather leaving
the bath house too soon, perhaps in inclement weather,
whilst his skin is perspiring freely, or his hair is soaking wet.

Again, it is not unusual to hear complaints that the
bath has induced considerable depression, or even
exhaustion, lasting perhaps several days; but here
again the fault rests with the bather. The bath must
be adapted to the strength of the patient, and it is
always prudent to take the first bath circumspectly, the
bather not staying too long in the hot chamber, and
undergoing the bracing application only a few seconds,
with water not very cold. It is difficult to point out
the precise time a bather ought to remain in the hot
chamber If delicate, and it is his first bath, he
should not enter a chamber hotter than 130 ° to 140 °
Fah., and should stay there only twenty minutes or
half an hour, or less, should he feel faint or tired.
The patient's sensations are the best guide; sometimes
especially if suffering from pain, the bath sooths and
eases, and then he can remain in the hot chamber an
hour, the first bath; but I repeat, he should at once
leave when he feels faint or tired. At first, the patient,
not seldom, on commencing the bath, fails to perspire;
in this case, he should be removed from the chamber
in ten minutes, have warm water poured over him, and
be well shampooed, and, unless he is tired or faint,
should then return to the hot chamber. It is a rule in
these establishments to advise even an old bather not
to enter the hotter chamber of 180 ° to 220 ° Fah.,
till the skin has become moist with perspiration;
though many disregard this injunction with apparent

impunity. Even if the first bath causes some depression, this need not happen afterwards, partly because the bather will have become accustomed to the process, and partly because he will know how to adapt it to his strength. Yet it must be admitted that some persons, even with every precaution, cannot take a Turkish Bath without experiencing much depression. Acute rheumatism and acute gout have been treated with these baths; but, as in most instances, the severity of the pain renders it impracticable to take patients thus affected to a Turkish Bath, a modified substitute for it, shortly to be described, may be taken at home. The acute pain of gout, it is said, disappears in the hot chamber to return soon afterwards in a diminished degree.

The Turkish Bath is particularly valuable in subacute and chronic gout, but, as might be expected, it is not in all cases equally serviceable. In long standing cases, in which the attacks have occurred so frequently as to distort the joints by deposits, the patients are perhaps liable to repeated relapses, and are scarcely ever free from pain, the efficacy of the bath, though striking, is less apparent than in milder and more tractable forms; yet even in these severe cases, the bath affords considerable relief by diminishing the frequency and severity of the relapses and by removing the pervading sensation of invalidism.

The Turkish Bath is perhaps more efficacious than other remedies in cases of the following kind: A patient inclined to stoutness, complains of slight and fugitive pains; the joints, but little swollen, are merely stiff and a little red and hot. The gout affects many

parts, often in succession—the joints, the head, the
back, and perhaps some of the internal organs, as the
bladder, etc. During an attack the patient complains
of *malaise*, and his complexion often becomes dullish.
The tissues are often soft and flabby, and in spite of
judicious diet and abundant exercise, the patient may
be seldom free from some evidence of gout, sufficient
to annoy but not to disable him for work. After one
or two baths the pains, the swellings, and the *malaise*
disappear, the joints become supple, and after a time,
the baths being continued, the complexion loses its
sallowness, the tissues become firm, and the undue
stoutness undergoes diminution. On discontinuing the
baths the gouty symptoms will often occur again to
disappear on the resumption of the treatment. A
gouty patient may advantageously supplement the
action of the Turkish Bath by drinking certain suitable
natural mineral waters.

The Turkish Bath is useful in the various kinds of
chronic rheumatism. A patient who, in damp weather,
or during an east or northeast wind, suffers from stiffness and pains in several joints, will derive much benefit from a Turkish Bath. The shoulder joint is often
affected, the pain and tenderness being frequently limited to a small spot.

Again, a patient without any previous history of
rheumatism, finds his shoulder set fast, is unable to
move it except to a limited extent, without great pain.
Here, again, the pain and tenderness may be very cir-
cumscribed. In such a case a Turkish Bath generally
affords great relief. Galvanism, too, even one application, will often entirely remove or greatly lessen the

pains and stiffness. Again, the Turkish Bath gives much relief in mild and chronic rheumatoid arthritis, and often retards the march of this disease. The bath often relieves lumbago.

Mr. Milton finds the bath useful in allaying the tormenting itching of prurigo unconnected with lice.

Should it happen that the regular Turkish Bath is not available, then one or the other of the following modifications of it may be substituted : The patient, quite naked, seated on a wicker chair, with his feet on a low stool, is enveloped in two or three blankets, the head alone being exposed, and a spirit lamp with a large wick is placed under the chair. In about a quarter of an hour perspiration streams down the body, and this secretion may be increased by drinking plentifully of water, and by placing a pan of water over the lamp. When the patient has perspired sufficiently, the blankets are quickly removed, and one or two pailfuls of cold water are poured over him ; or, if this effusion is too heroic, he may step into a general bath at 80°, or, better still, a few degrees lower. Dr. Taylor, of Nottingham, finds this treatment useful in obstinate skin affections, rheumatism, catarrh, syphilis, and in reducing stoutness arising from an inactive life. The instrument makers now supply convenient forms of the domestic Turkish Bath. It is far better, however, when practicable, to employ the Turkish Bath itself.

Dr. Nevin highly recommends the following handy steam bath in the treatment of acute rheumatism, available when the patient is lying helpless and irremovable in bed : A couple of common red bricks are placed in an oven hot enough for baking bread, and in half an hour, or a little more, they are sufficiently heated for the purpose. The patient's body linen having been previously removed, these two bricks are folded up in a piece of common thick flannel, thoroughly soaked in vinegar, and laid on two plates; one is to be placed about a foot distant from one shoulder, and the other about equally distant from the opposite leg, and the bed clothes are then to cover the bricks and the patient closely around the neck. A most refreshing acid steam bath is thus obtained; and the supply of steam may be kept up, if necessary, by removing one brick and replacing it by another hot one kept in reserve. When the patient has been in the bath fifteen or twenty minutes, the bed clothes and plates should be removed and *the patient instantly mopped all over very rapidly, with a towel wrung out in cold water*, and then quickly rubbed dry. Dry warm linen must be put on at once, and dry bed clothes must replace those which were on the bed previously. The under sheet can be re_ moved and a dry one substituted, by fastening the corners of the dry sheet to those of the damp one; generally very little difficulty is met with in simply drawing the old sheet from under the patient when the dry one follows it and is left in its place. The patient ordinarily experiences great and speedy relief from this bath. The exhausting sweats are usually diminished, and the necessity of opium much lessened. The change of the body linen can be easily accomplished by tearing the night shirt open from top to bottom, down the back. The steam bath and subsequent cold douche should be continued after the patient is able to walk about, as they contribute to the healthy action of the skin, and promote free mobility of the joints. After the patient is able to get out of bed, the bath may be administered in the manner previously described. The steam bath, according to Dr. Sieveking, relieves the pain and checks the perspiration in acute rheumatism, to a degree he has failed to attain by any other treatment.—*Dr. Sydney Ringer's Therapeutics.*

The Physiology of the Turkish Bath.

With the exception of a paper in the *Lancet* of May 20, 1876, by Dr. J. C. Bucknill, and another read by Dr. Cameron, at the meeting of the British Medical Association in 1877, all accounts of the Turkish Bath have been confined to general descriptions of the details of the process, and of the sensations experienced during its use. Except in these papers I can find no record of any attempts to measure, with scientific accuracy, any of the various powerful effects which it is universally acknowledged to produce upon the bodily functions. In the hope of determining by experiment the exact action of hot dry air upon man, I have for several years carried on a series of observations.

I presume that my readers are all acquainted with the details of a Turkish Bath. If not, there are many books from which they can be learned—notably that by Professor Erasmus Wilson upon the subject. Suffice it to say, that the essential part of the process consists in the immersion of the body in dry air at a temperature varying from 130° F. to 200° F., for a considerable time (half an hour to an hour generally,) and subsequent douching with cold water. The accessories of shampooing, etc., are non-essential.

Our power of tolerating very great heat, provided the air is dry, without injury or inconvenience, has long been known. Indeed, Drs. Forsyth and Blagden, more than a century ago, submitted themselves to a temperature of 260 ° F. (127 ° C.,) without great inconvenience.

All the experiments were made upon myself, invariably before dinner, say 4 to 6, P. M., and about two hours after lunch. They were performed in the spacious bath of the Arlington Swimming Club, Glasgow; and I may here mention, for it is an important factor, that this is heated by Constantine's system, which consists in an arrangement of stoves by which a constant current of pure air is drawn from the outside atmosphere, heated by passing through a species of oven, and driven into one of the apartments of the bath with such force that it traverses the whole suite of rooms, parting with some of its heat in each, and ultimately passing out from the last into the air. By this means not only is the air for breathing, but also the air in contact with the skin, constantly renewed, so that a layer of watery vapor does not, as in all baths heated with stationary air, soon cover the body, and convert the bath into a vapor one. The freedom from all feeling of oppression, even at very high temperature, experienced in a bath thus heated, is the best proof of the excellence of the system.

The temperatures at which the experiments were conducted, were generally an initial heat of about 170 ° F. for a few minutes, to produce diaphoresis rapidly, followed by a subsequent temperature of about 130 ° F., during the remainder of the time spent in the hot rooms. This, I believe, is the best system for habitual bathers, as perspiration, being once freely established in the hottest room, is kept active by the lower degree of heat.

What I set myself to investigate was the effect of immersion in this hot dry air,—

1. Upon the amount of material eliminated from the body in excess of the normal.

2. The alteration produced in the temperature of the body.

3. The influence upon the pulse rate.

4. The influence on the respiratory rate.

5. The alteration in the composition of the urine.

6. The composition of the sweat.

7. The arterial tension as shown by the sphygmograph.

We have now to consider the modes of making the experiments under each of the above heads, and the results obtained.

WEIGHT.

1. First, as to the amount of material eliminated from the body in excess of the normal. It is evident that to estimate this it was necessary to ascertain the exact weight before and after the bath, and the quantity of water drunk during the time. For this purpose I employed a beam turning with $\frac{1}{4}$ oz., when loaded with 3 cwt., with which all the weighings were done.

As the time occupied by the experiments varied considerably, I have in the following table reduced the totals to loss per minute.

TABLE I.

EXPERIMENT.	ACTUAL LOSS IN OUNCES, DRACHMS.		TOTAL TIME IN MINUTES.	LOSS PER MINUTE IN DRACHMS.	GRAINS.
1	60	0	60	8	0
2	38	6	55	5	38 10-55
3	22	4	30	6	0
4	35	0	55	5	5 25-55
5	24	4	40	4	54
6	24	0	40	4	48

This gives an average total loss of weight of 34 ounces 1 drachm in an average time of 46 minutes 40 seconds, that is an average loss per hour of 44 ounces— per minute of 5 drachms 53 grains.

The amount of water drunk averaged 4 drachms 44 4-7 grains per minute, so that the excess of loss over water consumed is 67 3-7 grains per minute.

Seguin calculates the average normal loss by skin and lungs is 18 grains per minute.

Now, all this material must have been removed either by the skin or lungs, no doubt by both, and I fear it is impossible to estimate how much passed off by each of those channels. However, it is a fact of great importance to know that by these two channels can be eliminated in an hour more than 44 ounces of the constituents of the body—not much less bulk than is normally excreted by the kidneys in 24 hours.

No doubt the amount of the solid constituents is much smaller, although by no means inconsiderable; nevertheless, even if we consider what is lost as pure water, it is obvious that the interchange of such a quantity of fluid in the economy must produce, or at least determine, important metamorphoses. In fact, the process may be fairly considered as a washing of all the tissues of the body from within outward.

TEMPERATURE.

Next, as to the effect upon the temperature.

The estimation of this presented some difficulty, as it is obvious that the thermometer employed must all the time be rigorously enclosed in the body, and no part of it ever permitted to come in contact with the hot air. To effect this there seems only two means available, its insertion into the rectum, or its retention in the closed mouth. The necessity of walking from a cool room into a hot one and back again militated strongly against the first of these situations, so I had an instrument constructed of a U-shape, originally with the intention of placing it on the floor of the mouth, with a leg on each side of the frenum of the tongue. When the instrument was in this position it was found to produce such discomfort that I was obliged to use it lying in the cheek outside the jaws. In this position all the readings were obtained. The thermometer was set, put in place, and the mouth closed in a cool room, the hot room then entered, the mouth being kept rigorously shut, and breathing being carried on by the nose until, after the lapse of ten minutes, the cool room was again entered, and the thermometer read and noted.

In this way, as far as possible, I avoided the direct action of the hot air on the thermometer, and I do not think that it can have been much affected either by the heat passing through the cheeks or from the nasal cavity. It is possible, although I tried to avoid this, that some small quantities of heated air may have entered the mouth from behind and affected the instrument. However, the regularity of the results obtained in many experiments militates against the probability of this source of error having produced much effect. The chart gives the average of a number of observations. I

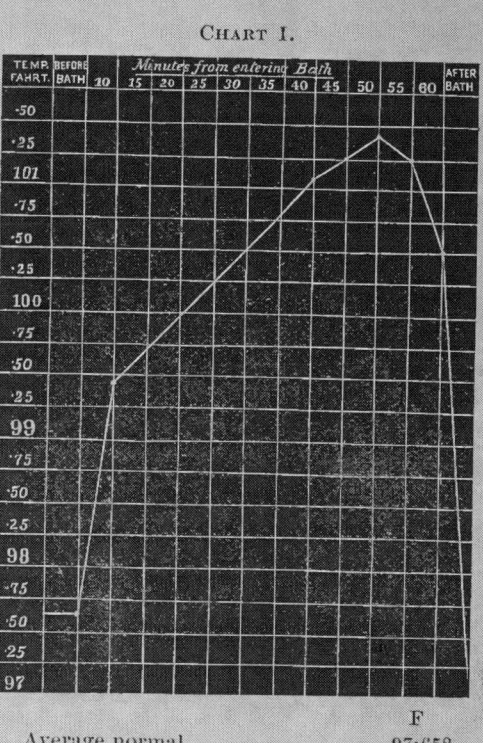

Chart I.

Average normal - - - 97·65°
" rise at end of 10 minutes, 1·6°
" highest point, - - 101·3°
" after bath, - - - 97·2°

do not, however, vouch so much for absolute as relative accuracy of the figures, since, from the peculiar construction of the thermometer, it is probably not to be entirely depended upon. As the amount of alteration, rather than the actual temperature, is what we wish to discover, this is of less moment.

Thus we have a rise of 3·7° F. produced by the bath, and this highest temperature was always reached at the end of fifty minutes. On the few occasions on which the experiment was prolonged to sixty minutes, a tendency to fall during the last part of the time was observed.

It is worthy of note that in the experiments described by Dr. Bucknill and made by Dr. Duckworth Williams, the rise of temperature observed was 1·7°, and, as the period of immersion in the cases recorded by them was always very short, this coincides exactly with my own observation at the end of ten minutes. As in Dr. Cameron's observations the whole of the thermometer was not enclosed in the mouth, I think the higher temperatures he obtained are probably due to direct heating of the instrument.

PULSE.

The pulse follows much the same course of temperature, but the variations are greater. Especially did the rate before the bath vary on different days. Besides, the effect of thirst was observed to be an acceleration of the pulse rate, which again fell after water was drunk. This was probably due to the reflex effect of the cold water, and perhaps somewhat to the irritating action of the too highly concentrated blood upon the heart

The following chart shows the average of many observations.

The rise in the pulse-rate during the first ten minutes was a little over thirteen beats The maximum, 116, was, as in the case of the temperature, attained at fifty minutes, after which a slight fall took place After the douche the return was nearly but not quite to normal on the average, but in one case it was as much as fourteen lower than before the bath. On this occasion the initial rate was high. I will again refer to this in considering the ratio subsisting between the pulse and respiration rates.

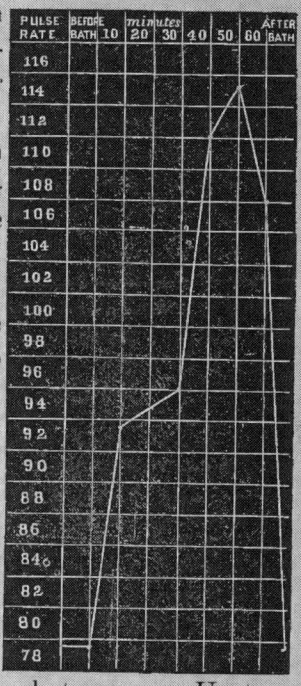

CHART II.

RESPIRATION.

In the paper in the *Lancet* referred to above, Dr. Bucknill's chief conclusion is that the rate of respiration is diminished during the stay in the hot rooms. Up to a certain point I have been able to confirm this result, as the following average chart shows:

Here we have a marked fall as the first effect, followed by a steady rise to a point higher than the initial, and after the bath a fall to near the number previous to the bath. This does not altogether coincide with

the results recorded by Drs. Bucknill and Duckworth
Williams in the paper referred to. They give the
average diminution in the respiratory rate as 4.2,
which closely corresponds with my result, namely,
a diminution of 4 ; but they make no mention of the
subsequent rise which I always found. This is probably due to the short time they kept their patients in
the bath. They, besides, merely state that the observations were taken during the profuse perspiration,
and not the time after entering the hot room. The
average rates of pulse and respiration before the bath
were in my observations—pulse, 79·4 ; respiration,
22·5. That is a ratio of 2 to 7, somewhat higher
than the normal. At ten minutes the rates were—
pulse, 92·5 ; respiration, 20 8 ; a ratio of 2 to 8·8,
which is nearer the normal ; at fifty minutes, 115·5 to
25·4 ; a ratio of 2 to 8·6. The well-known difficulty
of not altering the rate of breathing when counting it
yourself may have introduced error into these figures,
but on several of the occasions medical friends counted
for me. Their estimations nearly coincided with my
own, except in the initial rate ; and as my own result
was abnormally high, I have in the above calculations
adopted theirs.

SWEAT AND URINE

As the mutual relations of the constituents of the
sweat and urine excreted during the bath are the most
important parts of this branch of the investigation,
they will best be treated together. The method
adopted for procuring the sweat was the enclosure of
one of the arms in an india-rubber bag, confined round
the shoulder by elastic bands, and furnished with an

exit tube, closed by a clip. By this arrangement about 2 oz. sweat could be collected during an ordinary bath. The urine was passed immediately before entering the bath, and again after complete cooling. The sweat thus collected was found to have an average specific gravity of 1006·3, and to be faintly alkaline or neutral. The urine after the bath had a greater specific gravity (12 ° of urinometer) than before the bath.

I have to thank Mr. W. J. Mackenzie for the careful chemical analyses he has made of these fluids. From the small quantities I was able to place at his disposal, the estimation was necessarily confined to the principal constituents—chlorides and nitrogenous substances—which we presume to be urea. For the first of these the process he adopted consisted in evaporation with a little nitrate of potash, ignition to destroy organic coloring matter, and precipitation with silver nitrate.

The urea was estimated by Russel and Wert's hypobromite solution.

The mean of his results stated per thousand is given in the following table :—

TABLE II.

SWEAT AND URINE. IN 1000 Parts.

	URINE BEFORE BATH.	SWEAT.	URINE AFTER BATH.
Chlorides	5·68	6·05	3·65
Urea.....................	17 61	1·55	19·18

From this we see that the sweat contained more chlorides than the urine before the bath, and nearly double the amount present in the urine secreted during and immediately after the bath. Whether the abnormally small amount of chlorides existing in the urine (not much more than half the amount given by Vogel as normal) influenced this or not, further experiments on different individuals will be required to ascertain, and whether this diminution of the urinary chlorides after free action of the skin has any bearings on the well-known reduction in their amount which is found in pneumonia and other acute diseases seems worthy of clinical investigation.

The urea, on the other hand, follows a very different course. We have a considerable quantity in the sweat, and an increased amount in the urine secreted during and after the bath. The existence of urea in the sweat is doubted by many physiologists, and out of the three principal analyses of this excretion by Favre, Shottin, and Funke, Favre finds only 0 044; Shottin, none; Funke, 1·55, per 1000. The absolute identity of the latter with Mr. Mackenzie's result is interesting.

The amount of urea in the urine before the bath is about normal. The increase in the urine after the bath is probably due to the increased density of the fluid, and the high temperature which the body reaches—a temperature like that of fever.

BLOOD PRESSURE.

The difficulty of obtaining sphygmographic tracings in the bath was greater than I expected. I did not venture to expose a Mareys sphygmograph to the heat and moist handling necessary; besides, I doubt if it is possible to manipulate the smoked papers properly under the circumstances. The Tambour sphygmograph, which I devised some years ago, gave some fair results, but even it was difficult to manage, and the effect of the heat on the india-rubber membranes may have somewhat altered the tracings. However, I think we are justified in concluding that for the first ten to fifteen 'minutes the force of the heart beat is increased, and that after immersion for about twenty minutes it becomes feebler. This is shown by the diminished height of the tracing. The rounding of the summit and decreased distinctness of the dicrotic notch seem to point to an increase of peripheral resistance, and perhaps to the injection of a smaller quantity of blood into the vessels at each ventricular contraction. The condition of the circulation seems to be a great dilatation of all the superficial vessels, and therefore a diminution of the quantity contained in the heart and deeper trunks. This probably produces a faster action of the heart, as the observations on the pulse show actually took place; but it appears to the author that the necessary result of great capillary dilatation is increase, not, as usually supposed, diminution of peripheral resistance. No doubt the opposite condition, capillary contraction, causes an increase of peripheral resistance from the greater difficulty of forcing the blood through the narrowed channels; but in the case of dilatation, the vessels contain an immensely greater mass of blood, and this mass must require a greater expenditure of force to set it in motion, so that increased peripheral resistance may arise as well from excessive distention as from contraction of the capillaries. It is probable that up to a certain point this is counterbalanced by the greater facility of flow from diminution of friction, but I conceive that when the increase of the capacity of the capillary vessels is large, and extends over a wide area, the opposite effect is the more likely to accrue. This, then, is the condition brought about by the hot air, in my case at least.

The trace after the bath was absolutely normal, while that obtained before the bath was one of decidedly low tension.

CONCLUSIONS.

To sum up, it has been shown that a very large quantity of material can be eliminated from the body in a comparatively short time by immersion in hot dry air, and although the greater part of this is water, still solids are present in quantity sufficient to render this a valuable emunctory process.

The temperature of the body and the pulse rate are markedly raised.

The respiration falls at first, but afterwards is less influenced than would be expected *prima facie*.

The urine is increased in density, and deprived of a large portion of its chlorides, while, if anything, an increase in the amount of urea is produced.

The principal effect upon the arterial tension seems to be an increase produced by the greater rapidity of the heart's action combined with the dilated, we may almost say gorged, condition of the capillary circulation.

From these conclusions we may deduce the following practical observations as to the use of the Turkish Bath in medicine :—

Its most important effect is the stimulation of the emunctory action of the skin. By this means we are enabled to wash, as it were, the solid and fluid tissues, and especially the blood and skin, by passing water through them from within out. Hence, in practice, one of the most essential requisites is copious drinking of water during the sweating.

The elevation of the temperature, and more especially of the pulse-rate and blood-pressure, point to the necessity of caution in cases where the circulatory system is diseased.

Excessively long duration of the bath seems to produce more or less depression, as shown by the fall of pulse and temperature after fifty-five minutes. It is probable that the time at which this occurs varies with individual idiosyncrasy. In my case, it is accompanied by a distinct feeling, which I can only compare to satiety.

The great use of the bath seems to be the power it gives us of producing a free action of the skin in persons of sedentary habit, or suffering from disease interfering with fluid excretion, and by its means I believe considerable elimination of morbid matter may also be brought about. Besides, and along with this, it is an efficient means, if resorted to sufficiently early, of relieving internal congestion, on the same principle, and with much greater certainty, than the usual diaphoretics; and in rheumatoid affections not only does it act in this way, but by the relaxation of muscles permits of passive movements, rubbing, etc. (shampooing), exercising a much greater influence than they would independently exert.

PHYSIOLOGICAL LABORATORY,
GLASGOW ROYAL INFIRMARY SCHOOL OF MEDICINE,
June 1879.

HEAT AND ITS USES.

" *We have hitherto known nothing of heat as a remedial agent in disease,*" and " I do not know of any work where it has been referred to in the most distant manner."

It is astonishing that such a statement can be truthfully made respecting the state of medical knowledge on the subject, and more astonishing that scientific minds should have lingered for hundreds of centuries on the very threshold, as it were, of a most important discovery. For, since the days of Hippocrates, hot applications in a variety of forms, as warm water and vapor baths, stupes, poultices, and other contrivances, have been always familiar to medical practitioners. Still, hot air, *as now applied*, was never made available as a medical agent until the establishment the "Hot Air Bath" by Dr. Barter, while the experience that has since been obtained promises to effect a revolution in the whole system of medical practice.

It is passing strange that it should have been so, because medical scholars were familiar with classical antiquity. In England we have the interesting remains of the Roman Baths, and in Ireland they had the sweat bath in actual use from time immemorial down to the present day; while the customs of other countries revealed to us by travelers, ought to have instructed in-

quiring minds that an institution like the Bath could
not possibly have survived the decadence and ruin of
Empires, and been preserved through thousands of
years among divers nations in every quarter of the
globe, unless it possessed inherent properties of utility.

By experiments carefully instituted and conducted,
we know that certain beneficial effects follow the exposure of the body to the influence of Heat; and although
we may know little or nothing absolutely about the nature or essence of what we call Heat, still that does not
militate against the utility of its existence, or our application of it to practical purposes.

On the all-important fact, therefore, that we have
perfect command over the blood circulation, by subjecting the skin organism to the influence of artificial heat, the whole sanative virtues of the Bath depends. Remember that every drop of blood courses
through the whole circulatory system many times an
hour—how by subjecting the body to the artificial temperatures of the Bath we can bring every drop of blood
freely to the skin surface, and subject it to a purifying
process not inferior to that which it undergoes in the
lungs—how, by thus attracting the blood to the skin
surface, we can relieve congestion of the internal organism, and at the same time promote healthy nutrition in a manner otherwise unattainable. Reflecting
on these facts, one will readily understand that the diseased bodily conditions, the therapeutic power of the
Bath consists in the combined action of all these truly
sanative influences by which decomposed waste—a prolific source of disease—is rapidly eliminated from the
system, and blood purification, the foundation of or-

ganic life and health, rapidly and simultaneously effected,

Erasmus Wilson has admitted the ignorance of medical men concerning the therapeutic properties of Heat, and with equal truth he might have applied the same observation to cold, or indeed temperature generally. It is only a few years since the Medical Faculty have paid any particular attention to temperature as possessing any remedial properties in disease. But when medical men get an inkling of a *natural truth*, they are apt to pervert it—to mar its utility by allying it with drug practice. There is a tendency to rush from one extreme to another, and we now hear of specifics and panaceas, in the shape of ice bags, keeping a rheumatic patient in a bath of warm water for days, aye, for weeks, suspended between wind and water, so to speak, recommended by drug practitioners in conjunction with their own "*Medicamenta*," so wonderfully curative in themselves—" so wonderfully curative " that one of the most able Medical writers has said " that their medicines killed more than they cured " The general action of the " Hot-Air Bath " on the processes and functions of animal life—the sources and springs of vitality and health—there will be no difficulty in understanding its peculiar power and incomparable excellence as a remedial agent, in the various phases of diseased bodily conditions. I am fully persuaded, and fully believe that this remedial power extends without limitation over every form of disease—that there is not any known form of bodily ills over which the Bath is not capable of exercising at least a soothing, alleviative influence, and this, too, even in the most hopeless cases, where all the resources of Drug Medication are utterly at fault, or are only operative in torturing the sufferer to the grave. This opinion is not speculative—it is the result of no fanciful idea or fine-spun theory, but is based on sound physiology, verified by experience, while its perfect truth commends itself to the *common sense* of every unprejudiced and intelligent mind that will bestow a moment's reflection on the subject.

We do not claim for the Bath (as many of our opponents accuse us of) that the Bath is a grand panacea for " all the ills flesh is heir to ; " but, as we have said above, it can be employed with confidence in all diseased bodily conditions, for its action, even on incurable disease, must be beneficial as an alleviative. Before referring more particularly to some forms of bodily derangements, I propose to notice the prevalent professional and popular errors which obscure and mislead the public mind concerning the *nature of disease*, and the effect of drugs upon the same. I propose to say it in my own way, avoiding all technicalities and *Latin* terms ; and if to the classical reader it seems to lack scientific phraseology, I trust it will not be entirely void of common sense, as most Medical text books of the present day are.

Concerning the Nature of Disease,

AND THE EFFECTS OF DRUGS UPON THE SAME.

Although Physiology and Pathology have been successfully cultivated into useful sciences, the Profession as yet acknowledges no authoritative exposition respecting *the nature of disease*. The most discordant opinions still prevail on the subject, and the light of science has been turned aside, and the experience perverted to sustain the unphilosophical teachings of drug schools, which are now, as they always have been, based on speculative fallacies as to the cause and nature of disease. In order that I may not be misjudged or accused of prevaricating, I will show the deplorable state of ignorance in which the profession is now involved, by quoting from the records of the Harveian Society, of London. It seems a committee was chosen from the above named society for the purpose of gleaning some information about the nature of disease and the action of drugs. The proceedings of this committee are also highly instructive, and afford convincing proof—were additional proof required—of how hap-hazardous and murderous drug practice, as blindly followed, must necessarily be The medical journals, in reporting the first meeting of the committe, say :

" It was agreed to commence proceedings by taking up the following subjects for investigation, viz.: The Natural History of *Rheumatic Fever* and its Treatment by 1st, *Alkalies*; 2nd, *Blisters*. The Natural Course of *Acute Idiopathic Pleurisy* and its Treatment. by *Calomel* and *Opium*, with *Fomentations Iodide of Potassium* and The Natural Course of *Acute Eczema*.

" It was resolved to circulate the subjoined questions among the medical men of the United Kingdom : *Queries*—Have you found any of the following drugs, viz.: Digitalis, Cantharides, Chlorate of Potash, Belladonna, Arsenic, Quinine, and Tincture of the Muriate of Iron (as distinguished from the other forms of iron,) particularly useful in any special form of disease? In what form of preparation, and in what doses, are you in the habit of administering these drugs? and what results have you observed to follow their administration in the diseases to which you refer? Can you, from your personal knowledge, give any information respecting the use and doses of any drug, not commonly employed or particularly useful in your practice? or can you give information as to any fact in Therapeutics not commonly known to the Profession?"

Here, then, is an authorative declaration of the helpless ignorance, concerning diseases and drugs, which now characterizes the profession, after all the accummulated experience of centuries, acquired by physicking countless thousands to death. It is for the common sense of the public to judge of the estimation in which *physic and physicians* ought justly to be held in the face of such confessions of deplorable ignorance, made by the luminaries of the profession.

Rheumatic fever, pleurisy, and eczema are ordinary diseases, and yet, these physic-sages admit they are without any recognized mode of treatment, and want to know something about their "natural history" and "course!" and then look at the list of potent poisons, they send queries through the country to glean information concerning poisons they are, and have been dealing out daily, in varied doses, to credulous dupes, without any certainty of benefit, but the reverse; recklessly experimenting on diseases they know little about, and with poisons, too, of which they know less. No wonder, indeed, the celebrated Dr Bostock declared *every dose of medicine given is a blind experiment upon the vitality of the patient.*

The ancients, we know, referred all diseases to a special supernatural origin, and their ideas, actually, were not more clouded than those of modern physicians, and they were more simple and less harmful.

Dr. Hooper, in his *Lexicon Medicum,* defines disease thus: "Any deviation from the natural and healthy action of the whole system, or of any particular organ," in which, I fully concur, and have from the first year of my practice. Disease is, then, a departure, in a greater or less degree, from the perfect working of our vital organism which constitutes the state we call perfect health. Hence, disease is an effect ordained by the Creator to follow the exposure of the bodily economy to certain morbific influences, and is, therefore, subject to natural laws just as certainly as health is subjected. *God has left nothing to chance.*

Thus we arrive at a great truth—that, as the Creator designed the normal operations of our vital organism to be productive of health only, the *phenomena which we distinguish as disease can never be the legitimate result of those operations*, but must be induced by something that has interfered with, and impaired their natural and healthful action. Now, we have seen that the Creator has endowed the human organism with a preservative principle—the " *Vis Medicatrix Naturæ*," whose function is to resist the conflicting influences that tend to the decay and death of all organized matter.

Thus, we arrive at a second great truth—that disease, in its first or incipient stage, is nothing more than an excess of healthy action by the preservative principles to resist some disturbing cause. This is no new doctrine—no new departure—but is lost sight of by the profession, and not taught in the schools of medicine. But this great truth was taught by Hippocrates two thousand two hundred years ago, and was revived and reproclaimed by Sydenham, the " *English Hippocrates*," some two hundred years ago, and it is admitted by scientific Pathologists, that, *primarily, disease is a remedial effort of nature*. This constitutes the only rational and solid foundation on which a natural system of therapheutics can possibly exist. Correctly understanding what disease is, and knowing nature acts to preserve the integrity of her own organism, the only legitimate office of the physician is at once clearly and positively defined, "*as that of the servant and interpreter of nature.*" But such, I regret to say, is not the case, so far as my knowledge goes—(of course, there are exceptions to all rules)—but a large majority of the Regular School (so-called) Physicians do so magnify their own importance, and augment their influence, that it has encouraged mischievous delusions respecting disease, and their ability and capacity to " cure " it, until a credulous belief in their " say so " has become a popular superstition, transmitted from generations of dupes and victims.

In relation to disease, and *the true principles and the means of cure*, the most universal and lamentable ignorance prevails among mankind.

People generally consult their physician as those who are skilful to prescribe remedies that will *kill disease*. Many, indeed, seem to think that their physicians can *take disease out of them and put health into them*, by the direct application of *remedies themselves*, when skilfully chosen and applied, of its own intrinsic virtue directly imparts health to the body. This erroneous notion of course leads people to place implicit confidence in drugs. The result of this error, in the first place is, mankind do not believe that their own dietetic, and other voluntary habits, have much, if anything, to do with the preservation of health, or the prevention of disease. In the second place, when ill they expect to be *cured* by the sovereign power of drugs alone, and in the third place they are ever ready to run after those who are loudest and confident in their pretensions, and in this selfish world, open the door for unbounded empircism and quackery, call it regular practice or otherwise. Such a state of things is, no doubt, primarily referable to public ignorance; and by the way I may say it here and now, that my main object in issuing this " Hand-Book " is to educate the masses, to make them rely upon themselves to keep well, and when sick, how to get well

without resorting to drugs—but more particularly to
convince them that they need not expect that they
can atone for violating physiological laws, by closing
their eyes and swallowing "like a young robin,"
everything a doctor may put into their mouths : for
people educated in the laws of life and health, could
not become dupes and victims of the popular drug
system.

The great truth to be borne in mind is, that nature
works in disease equally as in health—the product (so
to speak,) of the perfect working of our organism is
health—the product of the imperfect working of the
same organism is disease. But most medical men talk
and write as if *nature* was only present in health, and
that something they consider unnatural was present in
disease. This is not a mere quibble about words. It
is a matter of deep practical importance, for remedies
are supposed to be given to *cure* disease. But the
term disease, being perpetually applied to *designate
diseased conditions*, it can thus be seen that drugs are
perpetually administered to *cure symptoms*, while the
*disease that produced those symptoms is entirely over-
looked* and unmolested. No wonder such remedies
fail! But the above facts are really not the worst
evils that result from such mal-practice, because the
certain tendency of such practice is for mere functional derangement to be drugged into *organic* disease,
as they often are, while the drugs swallowed may
cause *new* and more frightful forms of disease, that in
a short time become fatal.

The source and nature of disease being now scientifically and *rationally* understood, the reader is in a

position to consider the appropriateness of the *remedies* employed by the (so called) Regulars, as curative or palliative in its treatment.

Irregularities of the Uterine Functions.

Dr. Robertson, the Medical Superintendent of the Sussex Lunatic Asylum, England, says: "Insanity is a disease depending on, and associated with various functional disorders, and especially with the perverted nutrition of the organs of the mind and derangements of the uterine organs. The treatment of the pathological conditions consists not in the mechanical administration of specifics, but in the rational application of the principles of medicine to each individual case. The indications of the treatment here are, to restore the balance of the circulation and thus to regulate the secretions and the supply of blood to the brain, and so to restore the healthy action of the uterus, the skin and the brain. Experience teaches us that such a result will only follow the slow and steady use of remedies influencing the action of the heart and of the nervous system. Of such remedies, none are so powerful, or so certain as the Turkish Bath— and I find the continued use, in such case, of this remedy, will, through its soothing action on the nervous system, and the relief it affords to internal congestion by determining the blood to the surface, modify, if not cure the symptoms of the disease. In irregularities of uterine functions, which in young girls is often complicated with mania, I have found in several cases a cure follow the restoration, *through the agency of the bath*, of the healthy uterine action," and he goes on to say : " Setting the mental symptoms aside, I would here state, that if the bath had only this one remedial power of restoring suppressed menstruation, its value in reducing the ills resulting from our high civilization would be still great."

The above testimony, in favor of the Turkish Bath, is a short extract taken from a report made to the house of Parliament by a committee composed of the ablest physicians, appointed by Parliament, to investigate the workings of the bath in government asylums where it had been introduced.

It answers so well for a text, from which I wish to write, although I have had but little practical experience with insanity, yet it goes far to substantiate what I propose to say upon uterine diseases which have come under my observation during the past twelve years—names, dates, and details, of course will be omitted, so that only those who may see their own particular cases mentioned, will ever know who the patients were ; consequently, I violate no confidences. Among the hundreds of uterine cases that have been under my care, I do not call to mind a single case of failure (where the patient has faithfully followed out our instructions) in suppressed menstruation. Even where the general health had failed—and many cases where the patient had been invalided for months— and irregular for years. In one case of suppressed menstruation with severe constipated habit, where *dementia* was fully developed, a course of less than twenty baths, restored the patient to permanent good health. This was accomplished in less than two months time.

Another peculiar case of irregularity, was treated for several months, where *dementia*, at last, was the most alarming symptom. Her friends and her physicians had decided to take her to a private insane asylum, but some good Samaritan suggested to them the Turkish Bath—as the person had a sister in London who was similarly affected and was cured by the sweating bath — for weeks the poor girl would not consent to a trial. Said she had no desire to get well; that no bath could be of any use, etc., etc., but her mother and good friends brought her to the bath for days. It was a painful and thankless task, but after a few weeks treatment, the catamenial periods returned, and from that day to this she has been regular, and all the secretions normal—perfect health. She has been restored to her family and friends, and returned to her social position, where she had been before her sickness, the bright particular star. These two cases alone, ought to convince the most skeptical physician that it is a subject that should not be sneered at by the most *profound* regular, and that the question of heat and the diaphoresis of the hot air bath in such cases, are facts and realities which they never dreamed of in their philosophy, and they can not much longer shirk the responsibility. In uterine irritations, in all their different phases, the bath works wonders. The best feature of the bath, however, is that where the bath is used by young persons as a custom, (say from week to week) no such troubles will occur, for the general health is improved and all the organs of the body are kept in a normal condition.

The Natural Test of What Can Prove Remedial in Disease.

It is a fundamental law of man's economy, that whatever does not aid the purposes of nutrition, must, when taken into the system, prove more or less injurious. The functions and purposes of nutrition are the sole sustainer of life and health, and we know that the *primary* source of disease is mal-nutrition. Nature has thus supplied an infallible test by which to try all things that may be proposed, as remedial in diseases, —*they must be in harmony with the purposes of nutrition*—they must aid and sustain nutrition itself—they must conduce to its perfect existence and action—not derange and corrupt, thwart or pervert it.

Now, whatever does not assimilate with the human system—that is, whatever does not contribute to the purposes of perfect nutrition, feeding and sustaining vitality, must necessarily be non-natural to the system, and more or less injurious, and whatever is so introduced into the system, the vital principle seeks forthwith to expel; but its expulsion cannot be effected without an expenditure of *vital force* the inevitable effect of which is to leave the system in a *weaker* condition than it was before. Dr. Edward Johnson, of London (whose authority no one will dispute,) says:

" By introducing first into the stomach, and through it into the blood, certain acrid and irritating substances, called *purgatives*, the stomach, which was healthy before, is now nauseated, its lining membrane is inflamed, its nerves irritated, and its functions disturbed. Its peace and quiet, if I may so speak, is interrupted and broken. From the stomach the irritating substance passes by absorption directly into the blood, and thence by circulation into all the important organs—heart, lungs and brain—which become irritated in their turn, till, presently, that remarkable power called the conservative principle, which is ever on the watch, to preserve the living machinery from injury, takes the alarm, and a violent effort is made to free the blood from its poisonous presence, and its expulsion finally effected through the bowels."

Thus one of the most palpable effects of introducing purgatives into the system is a general disturbance of the functions of nutrition and consequent waste of vitality in effecting its expulsion. It is equally true of all drugs—of all non-nutritious substances that do not assimilate with the human system. All the organs of the living body have separate and distinct functions to perform. Each organ has its own power of protection, or in other words, its own organic instincts, not reasoning entities, however. To illustrate : Antimony, or Ipecacuana, given as an emetic ; the moment it enters the stomach, the organic instincts recognize an enemy ; it goes to work and pours out serous fluid to dilute and protect itself against the enemy, and continues to do so until the stomach becomes distended to a certain extent. When it can contain no more, then by spasms the contents are ejected by what is called vomit-

ing ; but it is not always the case. The organic instincts
of the stomach (as I have said above), not being reasoning entities are willing to throw it off by the bowels (any
way to protect itself), and then your beautiful emetic
acts as a cathartic ; the bowels, recognizing an enemy
eject the enemy it has just received from the stomach, often with fearful gripes and growls. Take the Eye, for
instance, to further illustrate the way foreign substances disturb the equilibrium of the system. A mote
or any foreign substance in the eye, the very same results follow—serous fluid is poured out by the glands,
the eye weeps, and usually, *if let alone*, will succeed in
washing it out and protecting itself against the enemy.
The same thing occurs when you get a sliver or splinter
into the flesh—the organic instincts come to the rescue
by getting up an inflammation, suppurates, and the enemy is ejected. Mercury in its different forms (the
most deadly enemy the living body has to contend
with), is supposed to act directly upon the glandular
system, simply because the glands show the *biggest
kind of a fight*, to protect themselves from their most
deadly foe. Hence the *fame that drug has achieved* in
liver and the glandular troubles. The most learned
and famous physicians never giving a *thought* to the
fact that the organic instincts of the different organs
act, and promptly, too, instead of their drug ! When
this fact is realized by the profession, and that the
" Vis-Medicatrix Naturæ " *cures disease* instead of their
drugs, they will be less anxious in *assuming* that their
work is far in advance of their *Creator's* (for that is
just what their assumptions amount to), when you hear
a physician say, " I cured so-and-so, and I cured Mrs.
S. of fever of a very violent type," when the probabil-

ities are Mrs. S. would have got well in half of the time, if left to good nursing and hygienic treatment.

In closing this article I desire to repeat, and I wish to impress it upon my readers, that drugging is opposed to nature, because, perfect nutrition being the sole basis of perfect health, whatever does not conduce to nutrition—whatever is not in itself nutritive, cannot be good for man.

Imperfect nutrition is not only disease, but a prolific source of disease ; consequently, what necessarily tends to render nutrition *more imperfect* can never be rationally presented as remedial in disease. There is *no proof whatever* that *any* drug exerts *any* remedial influence over *any* disease—whereas, as Dr. Wendell Holmes observes, "the presumption *always is*, that every noxious agent, including medicines proper, which *hurts a well man*, hurts a *sick* one."

Dr. Holmes also said, at the same time, and on the same occasion, before the "Massachusetts Medical Society," "*I firmly believe that if the whole ' Materia Medica,' as now used, could be sunk to the bottom of the sea, it would be all the better for mankind, and all the worse for the fishes!*"

There is more novelty and boldness in another theory that has been promulgated by a Dr Cotting, in a work entitled, "*Disease a Part of the Plan of Creation!*"

It must be a comfort to mankind, under the torments of disease, and reconcile them to all the evils of *physic*, to be told, that the fault lies not with them, for that disease constitutes a part of the plan of creation ! To have any rational meaning, this must imply that the Creator made the human organization so imperfect, that the necessary result of its action must be disease. This is an audacious implication of the Creator to palliate the errors of mankind, alike revolting to science and religion. The theory is physiologically false, and contradictory to experience. "Disease is *never* the legitimate result of the normal operation of any of the organs. The *natural* and *legitimate* result of all *normal* operations of our vital economy is *always health* and *only health*, and if disease is induced, it is *always by causes which disrupt those operations.*

Opposition to New Truths.

If the *Hot Air*, or *Turkish Bath*, so called, is entitled to one-half the credit claimed for it, why is it that the faculty do not accept it? Why do not the boards of health make themselves familiar with its virtues, (if it has any?) particularly as a sanitary agent.

We have been interviewed time and time again upon the above subject. In fact, the question is thought to be by those who ask it, a cold blanket—so to speak—unanswerable. For people say if there is any merit in the bath, they, the doctors, would be the first ones to embrace it, and prescribe them for their patients. Not so, at all. If we reflect on the proverbial inertia of the professional mind, or to expect them to admit anything which does not accord with their preconceived opinions, or commend itself to the accredited dogmas of established systems, we cannot be surprised that the "Hot Air Bath" should have had to encounter the silent indifference, or open hostility of most of the medical profession—more especially of its so-called heads and leaders of the regulars. The well attested therapeutic properties which it presented for their investigation were received, shameful to relate, with an ignorant, irrational skepticism, by presumptuous guides of medical opinions.

Yet these very men would eagerly welcome any absurdity in the shape of a novelty in drugging—they would accredit any speculative nonsense in the form of a theory to whitewash manifest imperfections in their *empirical* art.

And so it has ever been in all ages of the world—while those who endeavored to enlighten and improve mankind "have been those who have suffered most from ignorance, and the discoverers of new arts and sciences, have hardly ever lived to see them adopted by the world."

This is a truth that is written on nearly every page of medical history, and it is by thus looking into the proceedings of the past that we can fairly estimate the worth of medical opposition when it is directed in our day against any such innovating improvement as the bath. Take the case of Harvey, who is now held to be "illustrious," demonstrated to his class session after session before venturing to publish it—his grand discovery of the circulation of the blood—a discovery that reveals to us the admirable mechanism of our being, so wonderful in design, so harmonious in its complexity, and yet so beautiful in its simplicity. But when in 1628 he (Harvey) ventured to publish his great work, what was the result? Did medical men welcome and embrace so glorious a discovery? Not a bit of it. They scouted and reviled him and his discovery. Harvey actually become the butt of the profession. He was denounced as a quack and an imposter, and they called him a dissecter of " frogs and other reptiles," that he was cracked brained, etc. Harvey lost caste as well as patients, says Dr. Pettigrew, his biographer, and he further remarks, that the labor and application of twenty-five years were requisite before his discovery and opinions were accepted.

Sydenham, the most celebrated of English physicians, who has been styled the " English Hyppocrates," a man of great original genius, yet because he endeavored to elevate medicine from the depravity and corruption in which it was sunk, he too, was reviled and persecuted by those who considered they held vested rights in the *gullibility of mankind.*

Similar treatment was experienced by the famous French surgeon, Ambrose Pare, who proposed to tie the arteries in amputations with a silk ligature, instead of the then barbarous practice of seathing with a hot iron. So great, indeed, was the reluctance to abandon the cruel cautery, that nearly one hundred years passed before the first French surgeon (Dronis) taught and recommended Pare's method. Jenner, whose discovery has immortalized his name as one of the greatest benefactors of the human race, was assailed with all the envenomed malice his jealous contemporaries could command. What! said they. Vaccinate! use such a diabolical invention and transform the human race into cows and oxen? The drug doctors of London reported cases that had actually occurred after vaccination, (reporting the same for truths) that they knew of cases where the persons bodies were covered with hairs and protuberances that betokened the development of horns and tails—and in one case where a young lady had been vaccinated, (giving her name in full) was so brutified by the operation, that she would persist in running on all-.

fours and lowing in imitation of a cow. Even the pulpit thundered at him as a monster of presumption and impurity. A learned divine, Rev. Dr. Rowley, declared the small-pox to be "heaven ordained," and the cow pox and its use, a " daring and profane violation of our holy religion."

The College of Physicians not only refused to give Jenner a license to practice medicine in the city of London, but advised him to leave the city, for there was no knowing what an enraged populace might do !

The celebrated *John Hunter*, whose life was devoted to anatomical and physiological researches of inestimable value to mankind, eulogized as the greatest physioligist the world has ever known,. this truly great man was ridiculed, maligned, and persecuted by the leading practitioners of his day, who were incapable of understanding the nature and value of his profound scientific labors. Sir Ashley Cooper informs us that a famous surgeon was hired to write him down.

Sir Charles Bell labored for nearly forty years to elucidate the mysteries of the nervous system, but at every step his investigations were cavilled at, his conclusions disputed, and the merit of his discoveries imputed to others. The history of anæsthetics in our day, affords abundant proof, if anything more were needed, to convince the public that the profession have invariably been opposed to all innovations, and that those to whose labors the world is indebted for many substantial blessings seldom have reaped any benefit from them. We have brought these few illustrations of medical obstructiveness before the reader in order that a just estimate may be formed of the value of medical opinion when pronounced in opposition to any discovery that promises to be of advantage to mankind; also, to answer the question which stands at the head of this article.

Sir Ashley Cooper says, on this subject, "That persons who object to a proposition merely because it is new, or endeavor to detract from the merit of the man who first gives efficacy to a new idea, by demonstrating its use, fullness and applicability, are foolish, unmanly, envious and illiberal objectors, and unworthy of the designation either of professional men or gentlemen!"

Now, while I have not the slightest desire or ambition to write myself down a martyr, or confound my name with Jenner, Bell, Pare, Harvey and Sydenham, yet, the cases are not altogether dissimilar. Medical ethics, and the treatment received by the reformer or innovator from the medical fraternity, has changed but little for the last five hundred years—the same persecution, the same falsehoods, the same abuse, the same ostracism is practiced now as then. Wherever it can gain a foothold, of course, there are honorable exceptions to the general rule, but the profession, *as* a rule, are much like sheep, "they follow the bell-weather," and woe be to the poor fellow who does not keep himself and his ideas in the old rut.

To illustrate my meaning: A man may be honored and respected—popular, professionally and socially— while he moves in a certain groove, but let that same man introduce a progressive idea in medical practice— say, the Turkish Bath, for instance, as a remedial agent in disease—what do we see? He is ignored, in fact, ostracised professionally, and if possible, socially. His best efforts to ameliorate the condition of his fellow-man are misrepresented, and a wrong construction put to every expression he may utter, or act that he may perform—as much as to say, there are no honest men (professional) outside the regulars.

For the most part, however, the objections that have been urged against the Bath are of a very frivolous character and not over-worthy of serious consideration, but a notice of them, and a plain statement of facts, that the profession, as a rule—in all times, on all occasions—oppose all innovation in the healing art, if not in accordance with their own preconceived notions and prejudices.

Legislative Needs for Preserving the Public Health.

THE NECESSITY FOR BATHING INSTITUTIONS AS SANITARY AIDS, AND WHY COMPULSORY LAWS SHOULD BE ENACTED GOVERNING THEIR USE.

Nearly eight years ago I publicly predicted that the time would soon come when the Turkish, or Hot-Air Bath, would be introduced into many of our hospitals in this city. My belief was predicated upon the manner in which scientific men, especially in Europe, were experimenting with the Bath, and reporting their discoveries in such flattering comments upon its unexampled efficacy for the treatment of all diseases. In fact, that period of active empirical investigation, which was participated in by the ablest medical and philosophical minds in England, resulted in the enactment of three several acts providing for the voluntary establishment of public bath-houses under government supervision; and in pursuance of these laws several such institutions were so far projected as to secure necessary appropriations, leaving only the mechanical work unfinished. These provisionary measures were incited and pushed under the excitement of a threatened cholera invasion;

but before the intentions of the act were consummated
the epidemic abated, and, as is the rule, the public permitted apathy to defeat the excellent measure aroused
under the realization of their necessities. This pecu-
liarity of popular indifference after immediate danger
passes, has distinguished the world since history was
in its swaddling clothes. We observe its illustration in
cases of great fires attended with severe loss of life;
such calamities give birth to fire-escapes, and municipal
bodies are generally moved to discuss proposed ordi-
nances requiring the construction of additional safety
exits to all public buildings and manufactories. But
before the completion of the necessary legislation the
horrors of the calamity are passed, and the public
again resume their indifference, to be aroused to a similar sense of their danger again by the next great accident.

In the profession of *materia medica* there are certain principles, though very few, that are definitely
known, and of the laws of hygiene there is but a partial understanding; but it seems to be admitted that
the knowledge of prophylactic or preventive means for
avoiding disease are much better understood than the
principles of medicine that will cure; and yet, anomalous as it really is, the profession of physic in its
practice comprehends only the treatment of disease,
rarely ever the means of prevention—we may say
never, except under the enforcement of a threatened
epidemic. In our large cities we have provided, by
municipal legislation, dispensaries for the apportion-
ment of medicines to the indigent sick, and besides
these there are public hospitals in which the patients
are literally fed on debilitating drugs and nostrums,

because our forefathers treated the sick in the same manner hundreds of years ago. Nobody doubts the remedial agency of the hot-air bath—nobody questions the fact that its general use would arrest the development of disease, and save untold numbers of lives, which are now being sacrificed to the treatment sustained by tradition; but these facts seem powerless to change the vicious order of existing things, and, powerfully as they appeal to the intelligence of what we esteem, as the greatest civilization of any period, yet the hand of detention and ancient practice arrests our progress, and leaves us grovelling and dying in the slough paved by the bones of our ancestors.

While my prediction, made some years ago, respecting the public use of the Turkish Bath, has not been verified yet, notwithstanding the lethargic condition of our legislators, I still have an abiding faith in the ultimate adoption of that most potential remedial and preventive agency, especially in connection with our hospitals and asylums. Medical authorities, to which the public instinctively turn for consultation in all matters possessing an inferential novelty, are united upon the declaration expressed by the British Medical Association, that *" there ought to be baths of hot air and warm water in every city, town and village. No medical institution can be worthy of the name without baths, for disease is not cured by mere drugs alone."* Another learned medical authority, discussing the value of the hot-air bath, in a paper read before the same association, used the following terse and logical language: " We, up to this time, have always paid our doctors for curing diseases, not for *preventing* them; and, consequently, very little of this unprofitable, viz., *pre-*

ventive hygiene, has been taught in our schools, or is to be found in our medical treatises."

Considering with what universal favor and exalted recommendation the hot air bath has been received by the medical profession itself, is it not a pertinent and exceedingly important question, "Why is there not some legislation providing for the establishment of such bath houses in the asylums and hospitals, and in other places where the poor can receive the benefit of this salutary treatment gratis?" The duty which the public owes to the unfortunate must be acknowledged in provision for their care, and with this an obligation is created on the part of the community to administer the most effective, and at the same time least expensive means for the restoration of health, and the prevention of disease.

Looking at this question in a philanthropic and practical view, let us consider the inquiry, "What effect would the hot air bath produce, were it introduced in our eleemosynary institutions? In the first place to secure the most desirable result it would be necessary to make the management compulsory, *i. e.* every patient would be compelled to receive the bath, properly administered, as the exigency of the case might require ; nothing should be optional on the part of either the patient or attendant. These necessary conditions being observed, the results can readily be anticipated. In the place of drugs, the use of which can never fail exerting a deleterious influence upon the constitution of the patient, even though they destroy. the disease, would in a large measure be rendered useless. Now, if the bath will arrest the disease, per-

forming the salutary effects of the drug, without
entailing any constitutional injury, then it must be
admitted a great saving, and an inestimable benefit has
been obtained. The question is now reduced to a simple consideration of the remedial and sanitary effects
of the bath.

If the hot air bath possessed any of the characteris-
tics of undetermined novelty, if future experiments
were necessary to prove its efficacy, then it would be
the part of wisdom to defer its adoption until such a
time as its usefulness be demonstrated ; but it has none
of these features. On the other hand, it is one of the
oldest and best evidenced prophylactic and curative
known in Eastern Europe, and the earliest center of
civilization. But it is not necessary to confine its
proofs of value to the old world. Here in the United
States, thanks to the spirit of indomitable energy in its
combat with ignorant prejudice, the bath has won
its prize medals, and demonstrated its hyperion sover-
eignty over nauseating drugs and patent nostrums.
Confining its evidences of curative effects to definite
limits, we can say, without fear of contradiction, that
in St. Louis the hot air bath has accomplished such
wonderful cures as may well excite the earnest inquiry
of conscientious physicians, many of whom are themselves patrons of the bath.

This subject does not demand a learned medical dis-
quisition, since the period of its experimental existence
has long since passed. It is now upon that broad
basis of public necessity, with its virtues so conspicu-
ous, that it justly claims recognition by our state and
municipal legislators, whose thoughts and acts should
be tempered by the appeals of suffering humanity.

Here, then, is a rich field for active philanthropic labor. It need not be expected that local authorities or our executive administration will voluntarily assume the initiative in this matter, but much can be done by well directed zeal, to instruct them respecting its importance, and stimulate them to exertion. The machinery exists by which this great blessing can be brought home to those who want it most—the helpless in our hospitals and asylums—and the cost is insignificant; in fact, the cost involves economy. We trust, then, that a true spirit may move those who have the means and opportunity to take this matter up, thereby promoting a cause, the success of which may yet immortalize some spirit akin to that of a Howard or a Wilberforce.

INSANITY.

EXPERIMENTS IN THE TREATMENT OF LUNACY BY THE
USE OF THE HOT AIR BATH—SUGGESTIONS ON
THE NEEDS OF OUR ASYLUMS, ETC.

Nothing so excites the compassion of the race as insanity, that most dreadful of all ills mankind is heir to. The clouded intelligence can only be compared to a soulless body, wandering over the realms of eternity, listless, vacant, solitary; an incomprehensible mystery clothed within a panoply of horrible yet unconscious misery. Nothing is so deserving of a universal sympathy, and yet, with all our unctious solicitude for these most unfortunate fellow beings, their treatment, considering the apathy of the profession, to say the least, reflects no credit upon asylum management or those from whom relief is expected. I will not, however, withhold the meed of praise due many progressive intellects, through whose well directed exertions many alleviating influences and practical means have been adopted which have resulted in the restoration of dethroned reasons and the salvation of many who were regarded as incurable maniacs. For the slightest benefit accomplished in this direction, humanity in general should feel profoundly grateful, and be quick to bestow its distinguishing honors upon the deserving.

But that progress has been provokingly slow is too apparent. The study of mental diseases has not brought special fruits to the profession, and even when the pathological causes and effects are partially understood, the apothecary's aid has been, upon the whole, as injurious as beneficial. The question " why? " can hardly be anticipated considering the enfeebled condition of both mind and body of demented patients. Drugs, to produce an effect upon the disorganized brain, must pass through every capillary avenue in the system, leaving its deleterious influence, like the trail of a centipede, through every fibre, literally eating its way to the seat of disease. It is a well known fact, demonstrated by the profession hundreds of times, that in all patients suffering from any of the forms of dementia, the skin is harsh, over which a crusted exudation forms, which closes the pores and prevents a free perspiration. Since effete matter of the body can only escape through the spiracles of the skin, any poison that is given internally must exert a doubly injurious effect on the body that is already suffering from arrested perspiration. In this fact is found the reason why medicine produces so few favorable results in the treatment of dementia.

Some years ago the subject of hydropathic treatment was brought before the medical associations of Ireland by Dr. Barter who, in an exhaustive discourse, demonstrated its advantages so conclusively, that Dr. Power, Resident Medical Superintendent of the Cork District Lunatic Asylum, became so much interested in the treatment, that upon his recommendation the Hot Air Bath was introduced into the institution, first, as a matter of experiment. Dr. Barter was selected

to administer the bath, and the success of treatment
is told in the following report which was incorporated
in a lecture he afterwards publicly delivered.

" The first persons submitted to its influence were
much pleased with it, and were anxious to go in again.
Once in the week was the time at first appointed for
its use, which was gradually made more frequent, and
after about four months use of it I found seventeen
persons had been entirely cured by it and sent home to
their friends. The cases to which I allude were a long
time in the house, and *classified the incurables.*"

"After some months further experience of its beneficial action, new arrangements were made, which
enabled me to use it more frequently and more generally, and since then from fifty to eighty patients are
daily submitted to its influence, many for its remedial
action, but the greater number for motives of cleanliness. Even these latter are wonderfully improved in
appearance by its use, and have acquired the ruddy
glow of health, instead of the pale and sickly look of
invalids."

" Those who had suffered a relapse after having
been sent out cured, showed no unwillingness to
return to the asylum, and even asked to be taken
there at once, in order that they might get the bath,
as they considered nothing else would cure them. I
never have seen any ill effects from the use of the
Bath except a little nausea and a slight fainting in
a few instances, but after a bath or two, these effects
disappear."

Dr. Lockhart Robertson, the medical superintendent

of the asylum, says: "As regards the use of the bath in the treatment of mental diseases, I continue to entertain the most favorable opinion. As yet we have no specific in the cure of insanity, such as quinine is for ague ; and I for one, do not look for such."

Insanity is a disease depending on and associated with various functional disorders, and especially with the perverted nutrition of the organ of the mind, as well as of the genital organs. The indications here are to restore the balance of circulation, and thus to regulate the secretions and the supply of blood to the brain, and so restore the healthy action of the uterus, the skin and the brain. Experience teaches us that such a result will only follow the slow and steady use of remedies influencing the action of the heart and of the nervous system. Of such remedies, *few are more powerful in their action than the Hot Air Bath*, and I find that by the continual use in such a case, *this remedy will, through its soothing action on the nervous system, and the relief it affords to internal congestions, by determining the blood to the surface, modify, if not cure, the symptoms which mental diseases present.*

These few words on the use of the bath in the treat- ment of the insane would be incomplete, were I to omit to notice a specific power to remove the nox- ious secretions of the skin so frequent with the insane, and which in the asylums of twenty years ago, one could recognize as distinctly as the smell of a dog kennel, and which still refuses to yield to ordinary ab- lutions. *The Bath entirely removes this unpleasant complication.* The Bath as a remedial agent is grate- ful to the feelings of the insane, and which they do not, like other means of bathing or washing, associate with the idea of punishment.''

Dr. Power's interest in the results of the bath increased to such an extent that he not only made it a permanent adjunct to the asylum, but exerted his influence to extend the benefits of the bath to other similar institutions, especially throughout Ireland. In a subsequent report he states that, through the instrumentality of the bath, the percentage of permanent cures increased from fifty-nine to seventy-six, while .the death rate decreased one-half. Under his immediate supervision the bath was daily administered, and in certifying to the effects, Dr. Power uses the following language in his printed report :—

"The managers of the Limerick District Lunatic Asylum, in view of the beneficent results of the Bath, also introduced it in their asylum, and Dr. Fitzgerald, the resident medical superintendent, as well as Dr. Lockhart Robinson, superintendent at the Heywood Heath Asylum in Essex, where the Bath was also introduced, certified, in the highest terms, to the curative properties of the treatment. The interest extended until the *British Medical Journal* contained paper after paper from the most distinguished practitioners, all pronouncing the Turkish Bath an indispensable auxiliary in the treatment of the insane.''

Among a large number of other similar cases cited, illustrating the curative effects of the Bath, Dr Robinson relates the following in the medical journal mentioned :

" A patient was admitted to the asylum in February apparently in a state of confirmed dementia, restless and destructive, complicated with dropsy and albuminaria, and threatened with paralysis. Until the 10th of May following, he was treated with all the usual remedies, but in spite of these he steadily lost ground ; the delusions increased, while the bodily health gave way ; œdema of the limbs set in, and he was so weak that it was necessary to carry him to the Bath, which was first administered to him on the 10th of May. The result of the hydropathic or hot air bath treatment was that in six weeks, the patient, who was a carpenter, resumed his trade, and in six months he was discharged from the asylum, sound in both mind and body, and able to earn a comfortable livelihood.''

The Bath has also been introduced in the Colony Hatch Asylum, and Dr. Sheperd, the superintendent, pronounces it a wonderful success, and has taken so much interest in the treatment that he has written a learned pamphlet on the subject. In every place where the bath has been tried it has won the favors of its former bitter foes, and, thanks to the intelligence of the progressive spirits of the profession, it is being constantly extended throughout England.

Discussing this question in our own homes, why can we not have the bath introduced at our insane asylums? If it has accomplished so much in Europe, why not receive the benefits of its healing virtues in our own city? The terrible anguish of the unfortunate beings who rave and fret in their dismal confinements, appeals to humanity in such manner that to neglect them is a crime which shames the name of mercy. The cost is insignificant, while the promise is pregnant with good assurances ; therefore delay has no excuse for a back-ground.

Public officials are slow to move: but there is no proper reason for manifesting an indifference which bars the doors of safety against mankind. An agent at once safe, powerful, agreeable and economical is offered, fully tested by experience, and certified as incomparable in relieving various phases of this most terrible affliction. Is it creditable to the civilization and intelligence of our age, that an active philanthrophist should be wanting to make it available?

Turkish Baths for Lunatics.

The condition of insane persons in this State is at present receiving some attention from the Legislature. A few days ago, the State Board of Charities presented a report upon the subject, in which were included the results of inquiry as to the number of insane persons in the State, the proportion regarded as practically incurable, the extent of the provision already made for their proper care and treatment; and also, what further provision, if any, the State should be called upon to make for its incurable insane.

From this report, it appears that the total number of insane persons in Illinois is upward of 3,000, or about one in 846 of the entire population. It is estimated that eighty per cent., or 2,400 are incurable. There are three State hospitals, and two private hospitals, which, with the Cook County Hospital, furnish accommodation for 1,130 patients. The completion of the two State hospitals now building will add about 570 beds, making provision for a total of about 1,700 patients, leaving 1,300 still unprovided for, except in county almshouses and yards and private families. There are 640 insane persons in county almshouses, and nine in jails.

In the language of the report, the condition of the 649, last named, "is, for the most part, extremely unfortunate. * * * The diet, nursing, medical attendance and associations of the insane are horribly inferior and cruel. It is a common thing for the insane patient, of whom the keeper, more or less, entertains dread, to be shut up for months or years in a close apartment, unwarmed, unfurnished, and in this situation his wasting life is passed; often without clothing other than a blanket, or bedding other than a litter of straw." The report says further: "The confinement of insane persons in any county jail is, we believe, under the present code, entirely illegal, yet we have known such confinement to last, in one instance, seven years."

There are various other items of interest in the report, and, as a whole, the document is excellent reading for Lent. It is full of impressive lessons. Here is a matter concerning the most pitiable form that suffering humanity presents, and with all our enlightenment we are shown to be but little in advance of our barbarous ancestors in the amount and character of the attention we give to it. Humane and cultured thousands will crowd the church edifices to-day, and the services will be peculiarly solemn. Christian society will assume the garb of humanity and contrition in remembrance of one who suffered at the hands of man and devil nearly two thousand years ago. The memory of the forty days of privation in the wilderness is revived and perpetuated by the observance of Lenten customs all the world over. How fitting the occasion for calling to mind the condition of the thousands who wander year after year in the wilderness of mental death, and from whom the light of reason is shut out forever!

The subject is worthy of attention particularly because it presents a field for humanitarian effort most promising of reward. The question of alleviating the condition of the insane is not the most important matter in connection with it. The certainty that a large proportion could be restored to reason, if proper means were applied, constitutes the paramount demand of this subject upon the attention of Christian society. It is a shocking reflection upon civilization to assert that not more than one-fifth of these unfortunates are curable. The means are easily within the reach of the authorities, whereby the ratio of cures can be doubled, and probably still further increased ; and this can be done without any considerable outlay in the way of money or attention.

One simple and practical means for producing this result may be found in the introduction of the Turkish Bath in all institutions where insane persons are confined. The use of this bath and the benefits arising therefrom are not matters of experiment. The bath has been extensively used in insane asylumns in Great Britain, with astonishing results. From a report made to the House of Commons upon this subject, it appears that the Turkish Bath was first introduced in the lunatic asylum at Cork, Ireland, in 1861. During the next two years the per cent of cures effected was increased from twenty to forty, and the ratio of deaths was decreased in the same proportion. The report says : "The Turkish Bath is very tranquilizing in its effects. It is very agreeable to them, and many regard it as a luxury. Its salutary effect has been of a marked character. It fulfills all expectations." The resident physician at this institution, in a public address, stated that after a few months' use of the bath seventeen persons who had been a long time in the establishment, and had been regarded as incurable, were cured by it, and sent to their homes.

The application of the hot-air bath in cases of insanity produced by physical causes is strictly in accordance with the principles of medicine and common sense. The inaction of the skin and a disagreeable odor from the body are usually associated with these cases. The instances where the suspension of the functions of the skin as an excreting organ are not associated with the affliction as an important cause, are rare exceptions, except where the disease has been inherited. It is a well-known fact that the wives of farmers furnish a large majority of the cases of lunacy in the United States. This has been attributed to the immense labor they perform. Is it not more sensible to attribute it to the fact that their means of keeping the body clean during a life of toil are exceedingly limited? It has been demonstrated that the bath is a most potent agency in restoring the healthful action of the skin, and hence the beneficial results of its application in cases of insanity. It is believed that it has never been applied in this country, but sufficient is known of its beneficent action to warrant and demand its introduction, on trial at least, in some of the institutions where are now harbored the 3,000 lunatics in this State.— *Chicago Times.*

CONSUMPTION.

Theories of its Causes and Treatment.

One of the most interesting theories in regard to Consumption, or tubercular diseases of the lungs, is due to MacCormac, a name of eminent distinction among European medical authorities, his investigations leading him to maintain that this malady is caused solely by breathing air which has already passed through the lungs of man or other animals—that is, air that is deficient in oxygen—the inhalation of air already respired being accompanied by the retention of unoxygenized carbon, or the dead, poisonous carbon within the body of the organism. The effete matter he considers to be the starting-point in the fatal tubercle—that is, not that it is to be assumed as forming the tubercle itself, but as constituting the poison from which tubercular disease takes its origin.

The deduction which he makes from this, naturally enough, to the effect that the greatest care should be taken to secure an ample supply of fresh air, especially in cases where numbers of persons are obliged, by cold weather or other causes, to occupy a limited space together, and in which adequate provision has not been made for a constant supply of fresh air. In view of this, the predominance of tubercular disease in nothern latitudes is to be regarded as due, not to a tendency in the climate itself to produce such a condition, but, rather, to the greater liability of huddling together for purposes of warmth—although it is probable that a diseased condition or irritation of the lungs, in such cases, may increase the mortification of the poisonous material. MacCormac's investigations satisfied him that where, in consequence of the mildness of the climate, persons are induced to live a great deal out of doors, or where the houses are not closed up to such a degree as to exclude the external air, or prevent its free passage, this disease becomes comparatively unknown; he, indeed, encourages open windows and drafts of air, especially at night, if the body is well covered.

Substantially similar is the view taken of this subject by M. Kiofrey, of Paris, considered in its climatic relations. Knowing that post-mortem examinations have so frequently shown that nature, under certain circumstances, cures the disease, the importance of inquiring carefully into the nature of these circumstances suggested itself to M. Kiofrey as paramount.

Pursuing this investigation over an extensive field—comprising, in fact, France, Holland and Great Britain—the results convinced him that a cure was effected whenever thin and attenuated men changed their climate and habits, one or both, and in consequence developed a tendency to become fleshy; he considers a high northern and southern latitude as alike favorable—deeming all the temperate latitudes to be undesirable—and names our American coasts, say from latitude fifty-five degrees north to seventeen degrees south, as con-

sumptive latitudes. Concerning this, it is to be noted
that latitude seventeen degrees south is precisely the
point where the trade winds, relieved from their moisture by the Andes, produce a dry air. Natchez, in the
Mississippi Valley, is found to be a favorable point for
consumptives, yet the place has a very humid climate,
and the nights are exceedingly damp, the wind blowing
up the river, and bringing the dampness from the gulf.
Another fact may be cited as of general bearing in this
connection, namely: The coasts of Patagonia are lib-
erally submerged with rain, and the natives are repre-
sented as physically a most miserable race.

But, that a change of climate is really beneficial to
persons suffering with this disease, is questioned by
many eminent physicians at the present day—that, in
fact, climate has little or nothing to do with its cure,
and that if it had, the curative effects would be produced not through the lungs, but the skin. That a
warm climate, too, is not in itself beneficial, would appear from the fact that the disease exists in all latitudes,
with greater or less frequency, and among all classes
and conditions.

Thus, in India and Africa, tropical climates, Consumption is found to be as frequent as in Europe and
North America; at Malta, right in the heart of the
genial Mediterranean, the army reports of England
show that one-third of the deaths among the soldiers
are by consumption; at Nice, well known as a favorite
resort of invalids, especially those afflicted with lung
complaints, there are said to be actually more native
born persons who die of consumption than in any
English town of equal population; in Geneva the dis-

ease has about the same prevalence ; in Florence, pneumonia is said to be marked by a suffocating character, and by a rapid progress towards its last stage. Naples, also, whose climate is the theme of so much praise by travelers, shows in her hospitals a mortality by consumption equal to one in two and one-third, whereas Paris, whose climate is so often called deleterious, shows a proportion of but one in three and one-quarter. In Madeira, too, strange to say, no local disease is more common than consumption.

One of the most plausible points made by the advocates of this theory is, that, as the beasts, birds and fishes of one region usually die in another, a change of climate cannot, therefore, unless exceptionally, be beneficial to an invalid—that, notwithstanding the greater adaptability to climate which man preserves, the human constitution is not to be assumed capable of enduring absolute changes of temperature without being more or less affected by it, a change of this kind generally tending, indeed, to undermine the health. The African's sturdy health fails him in the cold of a Canadian climate ; both visitors and natives die of consumption in Madeira, and the constitution of European residents in India often, as is well known, becomes hopelessly shattered.

The investigation of this subject by Dr. Burgess, of Scotland, appears to have established, substantially, the above points, and in the valuable paper embodying the results of his inquiries in this field, he also combats the idea so commonly held, particularly by unprofessional persons, that consumptive patients, by breathing a mild atmosphere, withdraw irritation and leave nature

free to work a cure. Instead of this being the case,
Dr. Burgess contends that it is through the skin, not
through the lungs, that a warm climate acts beneficially.
When a sudden change in the temperature produces a
chill, cutaneous perspiration is checked, the skin
becomes dry and hard, and the lungs suffer from excessive action—being now compelled to eliminate what
should have passed off through the skin—an illustration of this being presented in the instantaneous relief
which is generally obtained through free perspiration,
where difficult breathing, or oppression of the chest,
has been occasioned by artificial heat. What is best
for consumptive patients, therefore, would appear to
be an equable climate—the fluctuations, not the high
temperature of a climate, being the source of injury
to be guarded against. The late Prof. Joseph Henry
was an advocate of this latter view—that is, he attributed the deleterious effects in consumption rather to
the amount of change in the thermometer at given
points than to the actual state of temperature. To
the intemperate changeable climate of the New England
States, the tendency of which is to produce disease in
the pulmonary organs, is attributed the prevalence of
consumption characterizing that region ; the only season
of the year regarded as favorable to those troubled
with lung diseases, in that section, being the month of
September and the first part of October.

One of the most interesting, as well as valuable,
contributions to this discussion is the address by Dr.
Schreiber, in which he takes the position that moisture
and temperature and barometric pressure are, for consumption and some other diseases, not the important
factors to be considered by medical men in locating

sanitarium, but that, on the contrary, these are but incidental to the more important question, whether the air of the locality is free from injurious organic dust and germs. He says the term climate, which is so much used, must be understood as meaning, above all, air which is pure, containing no miasma, no organic or inorganic mixture, in which, therefore, rain or snow occurs frequently enough to continually keep it washed and pure, the benefit of such a locality and air for consumptives being, of course, unquestionable.

IS MEDICINE A SCIENCE ?

To the Editor of the Globe-Democrat:

St. Louis, March 27, 1880.—It is but natural that the human mind in all ages, and especially as it rises in the scale of intelligence, should desire to understand the true nature of disease. This subject has puzzled the brains of the best thinkers in the medical schools from the days of Hippocrates and Galen to the present time. And remarkable as the fact may seem, the problem through these many centuries has remained practically unsolved. Neither the profound study nor the minute observation of any or all of the learned Æsculapians, be he "regular" or "irregular" (for then, as now, the schools were orthodox and heterodox), from that distant period down to the present century, has been able to fathom the mystery. Disease was something to be dreaded, but not to be understood. Frequent attempts were made to locate it in the system, but always without success; whether it resided in the solids of the body, or in its fluids, was wholly matter of conjecture.

Have the brilliant discoveries of modern times cast a glimmer of light on this subject? Surely, in this the nineteenth century, when science and art vie with each other for the mastery, when steam and electricity are working wonders to-day, which grow commonplace to-morrow; surely, in this age of discovery and research, we have a right to expect an answer to the old, old question, "What is disease?" Shall we get it? Prof. George B. Wood, M. D., of Jefferson Medical College, Philadelphia, says: "Efforts have been made to reach the elements of disease, but not very successfully, because we have not yet learned the essential nature of the healthy actions, and can not understand their derangements." Prof. Samuel D. Gross, M. D., a medical writer well known both in this country and in Europe, states briefly but distinctly that, "Of the essence of disease very little is known; indeed, nothing at all." Dr. Thatcher, author of the *American New Dispensatory*, says (of fever): "Its essential nature, or the approximate cause of its symptoms, is still a problem in medical science, both on the nature of disease and the action of medicines." Other authorities might be cited, but it is needless; they all lead to the following significant conclusions:

1. That the real nature of disease is not known.

2. That the healthy actions of the body are not well understood.

3. That the *modus operandi* of medicines (that is, the real nature of their actions) is entirely unknown.

4. That diseases, if cured at all, are not cured by drug medicines, but by a power within the system itself, technically termed the *vis-medicatrix naturæ*.

5. That drug poisons, instead of curing diseases, simply cause them to disappear (though even this does not always happen), and, in so doing, produce

other and more dangerous maladies. In other words, acute diseases are converted into chronic.

Certainly, the above "conclusions" do not afford a very encouraging outlook as respects medical science, so called. If this is the "progress" reached after these centuries, may we not justly conclude that, after all, the shadows of the dark ages still hang heavily about us?

"Medicine," it is said by some, "is a science as exact as mathematics, based upon facts which can not be disputed." Suppose, then, we look into some of the "facts." Before doing so, however, let us hear what is said about them by some very high authorities. Prof. Gregory, of Edinburgh, author of "Theory and Practice of Physic," says: "Gentlemen, 99 out of every 100 medical facts are medical lies; and medical doctines are, for the most part, stark, staring nonsense." What are we to conclude from statements such as this? Did Prof. Gregory not understand what he was saying, or did he utter the words without duly weighing their import? Suppose we take the pains to ascertain whether any of his confreres agree with him on this very important subject. Dr. Ramage, Fellow of the Royal College, London, declares that "It can not be denied that the present system of medicine is a burning shame to its professors, if, indeed, a series of vague and uncertain incongruities deserves to be called by that name." And Prof. Jamieson, of Edinburgh, regards "The present practice of medicine" as a "reproach to the name of science, while its professors give evidence of an almost total ignorance of the nature and proper treatment of disease."

Turning from the above excellent authorities, let us take a single quotation from that able and orthodox organ, the *Dublin Medical Journal*. It says, " Assuredly, the uncertain and most unsatisfactory art that we call medical science is no science at all, but a jumble of inconsistent opinions ; of conclusions hastily and often incorrectly drawn ; of facts misunderstood or perverted ; of comparisons without analogy ; of hypotheses without reason, and theories not only useless, but dangerous."

If these are the opinions of men that stand high in the medical profession, what are we to think of the profession itself? If the " shining lights " in the " science " of medicine have so little confidence in it, how can they, how dare they, commend it to the confidence of the people? A science which is " no science at all ;" whose practice is a " reproach to the name of science ;" whose " remedies " have killed more than war, pestilence and famine combined ;" remedies that " cure " by " poisoning the blood ;" by " diminishing the patient's vitality ;" by " producing other diseases !" Verily, the blind lead the blind.

But we were speaking of " facts " not of opinions ; not of mere assertions, but veritable (and we will suppose) " demonstrable " facts ; something that addresses itself to the senses. Very well, they shall be forthcoming. We must step warily, however, for the paths we tread are dark and mysterious. Medicine, it would seem, either as a science or a remedy, is peculiar and obscure. Prof. J. P. Harrison, an allopathic teacher and writer, says : " We do not reason on medicine as we do on other subjects." And in speaking of mercury he makes the following statement: "That it cures we know, but how it cures we know not." Possibly his patients, were they consulted, would reverse the statement, somewhat as follows: "That it cures we have reason to doubt; but how it cures is sufficiently obvious," as the following quotations from the self-same author ought to show:

"It (mercury) produces rapid sinking of the vital powers," has "very injurious effects upon the mouths of children — severe inflammation, sloughing and death;" causes "palsy, ulceration and disease of the bones;" it "irritates the heart and arteries, and invariably depresses the nerves;" it is a "most powerful subduer of the energies of life." "It brings on a most afflicting and incorrigible constitutional disease, which often defies the skill of the most experienced and enlightened physician to cure." "Sloughing of the cheeks has risen from washes and ointments" (of it) "applied to the head and other parts of the body." "Disastrous effects have sprung from these applications." It "inflicts incalculable evils on the patient;" "produces *cancrum oris*," (dry salivation, or canker of the mouth), the "most revolting mutilation of the face, foul ulcers on tongue, cheeks and fauces," "eats off the nose and the bony palate of the mouth," and "demolishes the very pillars of human health." Could devastation be more complete? These are "facts" for those who want them. If theory is called for, the writer has supplied it, in these words: "When we produce a mercurial impression to cure fever, we substitute the action of the remedy for that of the disease." Which, gentle reader, do you prefer? Perhaps it would be interesting to know that the

use of this terribly devastating drug was first introduced into practice by that prince of humbugs, Aure-
olus Phillippus Paracelsus Theophrastus Bombast de
Hohenheim, as he styles himself. This unprincipled
charlatan, who flourished about 350 years ago, burned
the works of Galen and Avicenna, declaring that he
had " found the philosopher's stone, and that mankind
had no further use for the medical works of others."

In another article I shall endeavor to show that the
dreadful effects of the " art killative " are not confined to one particular drug, nor to the " remedies "
of a single school.   Ex-Student.

Medicine Not a Science.

The question "Is Medicine a Science?" stands at the head of three separate communications, two in the *Globe-Democrat* and one in the "Only Evening Paper" of this city, and as yet no replies to either. In order to answer the question properly and understandingly, we must look up the best authorities (Webster, Worcester and others,) and see how they define the word "Science." Each and all of them say "Science is knowledge—a knowledge of law, principles and relation. The comprehension or understanding of truth or facts. Truth ascertained beyond a doubt. Philosophical knowledge. Profound knowledge. Complete and true knowledge. Science is *applied* or *pure*. Applied Science is a knowledge of facts, events, as explained, accounted for or produced by means of power, causes or laws. Pure Science is the knowledge of these powers, causes or laws, considered apart, or as pure, from all applications."

To sum up we find that Science, literally, is knowledge. Nothing more; nothing less. I take it for granted that all of my readers understand from the above quoted authorities exactly what is meant by the word Science. Let us now apply it to Medicine or Physic, as it is now practiced by the profession (allopathic,) and see how harmoniously they work together.

Medicine passes current as a science, and in popular
acceptance is identical with physic. Is, then, Physic
a science? So, indeed, physicians would have the
the world believe, but let us lift the veil, and look at
things as they really exist.

"*Anatomy*," says Richerland, "is the science of organization. It deals with the apparatus, the instruments in that laboratory in which the chemistry of
life is carried on." Hence the peculiar province
of Anatomy is the examination, by dissection, of the
organs of animal life. "Strictly speaking, structure
alone is learned by dissection. The vital properties of
organic textures, and the functions of organs are found
out by observation." Anatomy, therefore, has a solid
foundation, and is truly a science of *facts*. Consequently it is the only basis on which sound medical
knowledge can rest.

Surgery, in the narrow barbaric sense that prevailed
in ages of ignorance, means hand-work, and implies
the employment of instruments, and the use of topical
remedies merely, in the treatment of disease. Such
was the ignoble sphere assigned to Surgery during the
dark ages of semi-civilization, extending even to the
end of the eighteenth century.

Its proper sphere will be noticed in due course; at
present it is sufficient to observe that, while it is based
on a thorough knowledge of Anatomy, general and
morbid, it also draws inspiration from whatever tends
to throw light on the varied and complicated functions
of vitality. It was by thus estimating aright the true
province of Surgery, that the illustrious John Hunter

succeeded in raising it "above the servility of a mechanical art to a science of the highest order."

Physiology is the science of normal or healthy life, and has an intimate alliance with, or rather a necessary dependence on, Anatomy, inasmuch as it deals with the whole phenomena of our organization in its natural state, and with the laws or principles in accordance with which they are manifested, and by which all the functions of structure are governed.

Physiology, consequently, has no practical value outside the domain of fact. It has nothing to do with speculative fancies, and it never can err while it keeps within the sphere of legitimate induction from the incontestible phenomena of nature.

Pathology is exactly the reverse of Physiology. It embraces the phenomena of abnormal or diseased conditions, and, therefore, is largely dependent on morbid anatomy. Still, in *diagnoses*, or in the art of discerning the distinctions of disease, can only be acquired as the result of observation, based on a profound knowledge of Pathology ; and the reason why so many fatal mistakes are constantly occurring in practice—misjudging effects for causes and treating symptoms only, instead of comprehending the true source of abnormal changes, is, that a lamentable ignorance of Pathology is a characteristic of medical practitioners generally.

Hygiene, or the art of preserving health, it will thus be seen, is necessarily based on a correct knowledge of Physiology. A knowledge of the laws by which normal or healthy life is governed, necessarily makes us acquainted with the conditions essential to its maintenance, while we are also led to comprehend how the violations of the conditions cause a disturbance of natural action which, when manifested in whatever form, or with greater or lesser intensity, constitutes what is commonly termed disease. Hygiene, therefore, rightly understood in a truly comprehensive sense, includes mind and body, and thus, in reality, embraces Biology, or the Science of Life.

Therapeutics is opposed to Hygiene, in so far as it contemplates the derangement of natural health. Its perfection consists in properly treating abnormal conditions, in checking the aberrations of disordered functions, and in contributing towards the restoration of natural action. Its chief duty, consequently, is to aid the *vis medicatrix naturæ*, or the principle of self-preservation with which Providence has beneficially endowed all organized creation. The *Healing Art*, as it is called, is, therefore, only another name for Therapeutics, but, correctly speaking, "art" never yet healed or cured any disease, while the supposition, absurd and unscientific, that "art" does heal or cure, has been, and still continues to be, a most fruitful source of error and suffering. All mere "art" can do, at best, though sustained by the most profound medical knowledge, is to remove foreign elements that interfere with normal action, and supply natural aids that may be wanting, and thus assist to re-establish those conditions which sound physiology teaches are essential to health—the *vis medicatrix naturæ*, the preservative principle of animal life, *alone* heals and cures. Hence, a rational system of Therapeutics can never be based on what is, in any degree, *speculative*, but must necessarily rest on a knowledge of *facts* obtained by the study of Physiology, and accurate observation of the varied phenomena of nature as manifested in health and disease. Just as the most profound knowledge of Anatomy, through the basis of Surgery, never yet, of itself, made a skilful and accomplished surgeon, so an equally profound knowledge of Pathology, or of diseased conditions, never yet made, of itself, a skilful therapeutist. The essential condition is, that all *theory* must be discarded, and pathological knowledge applied in strict consistency with physiological truth. This strikes at the very root of all systems of mere physic which have tortured humanity, because all have been based on speculative and unstable theory—not on the facts of nature. Hence, a physician may be, and often is, a very learned pathologist, very skilful in diagnoses, and yet, as a practitioner, nothing more than the servile follower of some empirical mode of treatment— the dupe himself, and unconsciously often so, of false doctrines, erroneous teaching, and imperfect mental training.

This makes up the sum total of all that can be deemed absolutely scientific and certain in medicine, and it will be observed that all this knowledge is essentially knowledge of *facts* derived from diligent observation and study of nature, consequently, has no relation whatever with anything that is merely theoretical, speculative or problematical. Thus considered, what then becomes of the popular idea concerning medicine and the medical profession? Where is the place for the mere physician to occupy who deals in drugs? What scientific, natural and rational basis has he to rest on as a practitioner?

Eliminate anatomy, physiology and pathology from what—among the ill-informed and unreflective of all classes—passes for "medical science," and honestly consider what remains behind. What, indeed, but the apothecary under the designation of a "physician," with his pestle and mortar, still and crucible, for the preparation of pernicious compounds, unnatural and poisonous concoctions, recommended, unchallenged and unexplained, by crude theories and speculative fallacies unworthy of this scientific age, and all at eternal enmity with human health, happiness and life!

Bearing in mind, then, the essential distinction between medicine as a *science* and physic as an *art*, it will be understood at once that it was not the former, as based on the demonstrative facts of Anatomy, Physiology, and Pathology, that the eminent Sir Astley Cooper contemplated when he deliberately said: "The science of medicine is founded on conjecture and improved by murder." It was clearly physic, or drug medication that he referred to.

It was also of medicine, as identified with the pernicious art of drugging, that the celebrated Magendie spoke, when addressing his students. He said: "Gentlemen, medicine is a *great humbug*. I know it is called science. Science, indeed! It is nothing like science. Doctors are merely empirics, when they are not charlatans!"

In the same spirit of candor the *Dublin Medical Journal* said: "Assuredly the uncertain and most unsatisfactory art that we call medical science is no science at all, but a jumble of inconsistent opinions;

of conclusions hastily, and often inaccurately drawn ; of facts misunderstood or perverted ; of comparisons without analogy ; of hypotheses without reason, and theories not only useless, but dangerous.''

In even more emphatic terms an esteemed author, Dr. Mason Good, wrote : '' The science of medicine is a *barbarous jargon*, and the effects of our medicines on the human system in the highest degree uncertain, except, indeed, that they have destroyed more lives than war, pestilence and famine combined.''

There can be nothing *uncertain* in science, and hence the *Medical Times* admitted that '' a *scientific* as distinguished from an *empirical* treatment of disease (by drugs) is an idle dream.'' And the reason of this may be gathered from the clever author, Dr. Ridge, who frankly says : '' That medicines, administered with the best intentions, and according to all rules of art by the profession itself, as well as by all classes on their own responsibility, aggravate the disease, and suffering is too clear to need any illustration.'' Even the *Lancet* has had its faith shaken in '' Physic as a Science.''

The progress of *true* medical science has greatly qualified our estimate of the value of mere drugs in the treatment of disease. It has shown that in medicine, as in politics, the best course is that of non-intervention.

The conclusion is, therefore, irresistible—that Anatomy, Physiology and Pathology, as based on demonstrative facts, can alone be regarded as composing medical science. Hence, an eminent authority, Sir Richard Owen, Professor of Anatomy to the Royal

College of Surgeons, London, in addressing the students of St. Mary's Hospital, Paddington, at the distribution of prizes in 1865, said: "Anatomy, Physiology and Pathology, all three bodies of doctrine worthy of the name of sciences, must be cultivated—if possible, mastered—as the indispensable basis on which a lasting superstructure of a true science of medicine can be raised." M. D.

AN HONEST CONFESSION.

Dr. J. L. W. Thudichum, Professor of Chemistry and Surgery in Grosvenor Place Medical College, London, does justice to the "Hot-Air Bath" in an address before the "London Medical Society," and published in their transactions. We publish a part of it—all we have space for—and hope it will be read by our Physicians and the public without prejudice:

GENTLEMEN OF THE SOCIETY:—We find ourselves unexpectedly in the startling position of having a most powerful, and, at the same time, the most simple agent for the preservation of health and restoration of well-being offered for our acceptance. It is not a discovery of science which we have before us; that boast of our days was blind to the uses of hot air as a means of comfort and health. It is a practice handed down to us from the early days of mankind; from those times when little was said, less was written, but all is done that is essential to the well-being of man. Science has not preserved for us an application known to every people on the globe before our era; nor has it been instrumental in teaching the West that practical tradition which that natural and simple people of the East—the Turks—had the good sense and justice to preserve intact in the condition in which they received it. Scores of travelers have given elaborate descriptions of this

institution; numbers of our own body now boast of
having had experience of the Thermæ in the land of its
last refuge. Yet to none of them is it as much as a
matter of surprise, much less of shame, not to have
utilized at once their experience. The blind did not see,
the seed fell among thorns. The simple discovered,
the simple preserved; one single man taught the West,
and in the West it was again the simple who accepted
the gift. How different was the bearing of the educated, the scientific, or even the prominent men of our
own society; anterior conclusions sealed their understanding, and barred their courage, even, from repeat-
ing those trials which the experimental mind of former
centuries has left for their guidance. They had not
the candor to see and try for themselves, and judge
according to the evidence, but denounced as dangerous
and fatal what meets every simple mind as safe, agreeable and soothing. The short space of ten years has
sufficed to exhibit the absurdity of these unfounded
denunciations.

For ten years the medical press, particularly that
publicication which is now so zealous in the multiplica-
tion of letters on what has, in spite of its attempted suppression, become a stirring topic in the world, ignored
an application upon which the scribes behind the scenes
now have the hardihood to claim the reservation of a
final judgment.

In the presence of such unprecedented circumstances,
what conduct is it the duty of the true followers of
science to adopt? By what line of action can the physician reconcile the part of his art to his present duty
to his art and to mankind? How can he do justice to
truth?

By that act which must precede every reformation;
by a candid renunciation of all errors of the past—of
all anterior knowledge and conclusions; by the resolu-
tion not to weave the new knowledge into the tissue of
his former errors, theories and practice; by becoming
a child in science, and acquiring new powers of per-
ception. If we are to wait these 500 years before
we know anything about the Bath, if we are to learn
in our life-time the value and the nature of the Thermæ,
the event will be announced by the figure of a man
standing up by himself; after having dropped alike the
clouts and finery of preconceived notions, making
renunciation, making confession, and starting with
freedom on the new career of experiment—the Beacon
of the human frame—to accomplish the *opus magnum*
of Pathology.

By the experimental process, obtaining results which
are themselves instruments available to every hand, so
as to make science the hand-maid of daily practice, I
have made that renunciation in full; and if I claim to
be honest by pointing my finger in the direction
of error, and by denouncing false principles of action
and modes of thinking, I am no less inviting you to
participate in the benefits of such an act, by imposing
it upon yourselves. United we shall meet the future,
and exhibit to the world such an imposing spectacle of
seriousness of purpose and truthfulness of mind, and
a harvest of success, that there shall not be the like,
at least, while ten generations preserve the love of our
memory

The discovery that was lost and has been found again,
is this, in the fewest possible words, the application of

hot air to the human body. It is not wet air, nor damp air, nor vapory air; it is not vapory in any shape or form whatever. It is an immersion of the whole body in hot common air. No sooner had I ascertained that a person had returned comforted from such an application, than I determined upon experiment and study. I derived knowledge of new truths and confirmation of former assertions. I saw fallacies exposed, and was startled to sadness. I saw the sick healed and the suffering comforted. I saw a new enjoyment added to the few that life possesses, and saw it within the reach of all. I brought away a heavy load of private gain, in the exchange of a delicate lung and a sensitive skin, for health, strength, and hopeful existence. As a physician, I felt placed in my hands the most powerful and certain, and at the same time, the most agreeable therapeutic agent in existence. A new day of the art of healing had dawned on the horizon, which Hippocrates claimed as an honor to have taught physicians I felt they were now being taught again; and I opened my ear to the teachers and the teachings. They are great and joyful, and their truth is patent to every eye. And I can enjoy them, and perhaps, multiply them, with an easy conscience, as I have closed accounts with the past, and have a clear scope of mind for future experience.

Turkish Baths vs. Arkansas Hot Springs.

Much has been written, and more said, in regard to
the invaluable properties of the Arkansas Hot Springs
as a remedial agent. Invalids, from all sections of the
country, flock to the Hot Springs with every variety
of disease, and I am informed by the resident physician that all are more or less benefited, and many rad-
ically cured, where all other known means had failed.
The question very naturally aries in the minds of those
who are willing to search for new truths—what brings
about these wonderful cures? It is evident to all who
think for themselves, that it is not the mineral properties of the spring water, for the analysis of the
water shows it to be as pure as distilled water, or
nearly so, notwithstanding they have the arsenic, sul-
phur and alum springs ; consequently, we must at once
come to the conclusion that it is the "diaphoresis,"
or sweating, caused by the heat of the water, rather
than by its properties. Of course, change of air,
change of diet, freedom from care and business per-
plexities have much to do with the cures, yet facts go
far to prove that the sweating process is the great
secret of the cures. The largest class of drugs used
by the profession are known as diaphoretics or sudo-

rifies, and are used more generally than any other medicines, but at the same time they are the most uncertain in their operation, and, I may safely add, the most pernicious. Now, I claim (and my experience will bear me out in what I say) that h eat stands mountains high above any and all diaphoretics as a cure in all kinds of diseased action, for precisely the same results can be brought about with heat without the injurious, and sometimes fatal, effects of diaphoretics. Now, if moist heat or steam is capable of equalizing the circulation, removing obstructions, relieving congestions, stimulating the circulation, and calling into action the secreting and excreting organs, how much better is the application of the pure dry heat of the " Turkish Bath." When I speak of the " Turkish Bath " I do not include those so-called Turkish baths gotten up by every adventurer, dubbing themselves Professors, Doctors, or what not—not knowing the first principles of Physiology, or the laws of health. A bath with intense heat, poor ventilation, is no Turkish Bath, and the public should not judge *the* Bath by such shams. Dry heat can be endured at a much higher temper ature than moist heat, while steam or hot water can only be endured at 110 ° or 115 ° at the highest : the hot air bath can be taken as high as 150 ° with comfort, and many take it much higher. I have taken one in New York at 250 ° with the happiest results. Hot air favors evaporation : moist heat does not. Dry heat favors absorption of oxygen ; moist heat prevents it. Dry hot air invites the blood to the surface, causing profuse perspiration ; vapor heat condenses upon the body and prevents free perspiration. A person with ordinary judgment knows this, by the acceleration of the heart's action. In a steam bath, many really think they are sweating, when it is nothing but the condensed vapor pouring off of them. The Hot Air or Turkish Bath of our city commends itself to all, especially to invalids. I hold that it is, physiologically speaking, far ahead of the Arkansas Hot Springs as a remedial agent, in any and all diseases, for the reasons above stated. Give the Turkish Bath half the chance you do the Arkansas Hot Springs—that is, by attending to them as you would do when you go to the Springs, and you will find that my words will more than prove true. You will then save a hard and expensive journey, w'll retain all your home comforts. The accommodations of the bath in our own city are far superior to those in the wilds of Arkansas, and last, but not least, a competent physician, of long experience in the practice of medicine, gives his entire time and advice to his patrons, and his accomplished wife her time, during the ladies' hours, free of charge. We hope, with Dr. Adams, soon to see a Turkish Bath introduced into our city hospital and insane asylum. Who will be the happy man (physician or layman) that will immortalize his name by being instrumental in bringing about a consummation so devoutly to be wished?

A FRIEND OF THE BATH.

The Difference Between Steam Heat and Fire Heat.

Mr. Rohrer, of this city, who beside being engaged in other enterprises, is a manufacturer of acid phosphate of lime, in which last undertaking he has heroically battled with the whims of chemical affinities till he can show about $10,000 on the wrong side of the ledger. In the course of attaining to this loss and a corresponding advance toward perfection in the process, Mr. Rohrer has discovered some peculiar facts, chief among which is that there is a chemical difference between steam heat and fire heat at the same temperature. The original ingredients—bone ash, starch and acid—are mixed together. It is then desirable to thoroughly dry this mixture, which goes into the drying room in small chunks preparatory to being ground to flour in the mills. With steam heat the pieces become coated with a glutinous substance that effectually closes the pores against the exit of internal moisture; hence the mixture can not be ground except with great difficulty and loss. With fire heat—heat given off directly from a furnace—these difficulties are not encountered. It might be suggested that there were leaks in the steam pipes, liberating steam and moistening the atmosphere. The starch in the mixture having a great affinity for moisture would thus naturally form a glutinous coating on the lumps. But there were no leaks, and to all human observation the air was perfectly dry, without the slightest humidity. The drying-room contained 2,500 feet of steam pipe, all exposed to plain view, and gave off more heat than was necessary, so that the system had to be throttled. After losing ton upon ton of material, the pipe system was torn out, and a huge furnace made of boiler plate, forty-two inches in diameter and seven feet high, properly jacketed, was substituted. No trouble is now had from the drying. Will some of our honored contemporaries offer an explanation of this phenomenon? We have been raised in that old school wherein is taught that a given number of degrees of temperature is the same in ordinary atmospheric air in its physical and chemical attitude, regardless of the source.

The above article was clipped from a Boston paper some few weeks since, and it occurred to me that it was one of the best proofs in favor of "Hot Air Bathing" as compared with vapor or heat radiated from steam pipes, that I have ever seen advanced by any authority, but I have ever contended that there was a vast difference between the two, in favor of the dry heat. Any one at all acquainted with "Hot Air Bathing," will see at once the great importance of this distinction when they reflect that in one case the body is surrounded by dry, hot air, which must favor the exosmosis of the watery portion of the blood through the coats of the cutaneous capillaries, and the endosmosis of oxygen, and at the same time favor evaporation. While in the other case, the body is surrounded by vapor, which would be absorbed in place of oxygen, while evaporation would be checked.

In the one case you have exosmosis of fluid and absorption of oxygen; in the other case, you have neither.

This explanation fully accounts for the glutinous coating upon the skin of bathers, when they first enter a hot room heated by steam pipes or vapor. I should not expect as favorable results in the treatment of diseases with vapor, (especially, in chronic cases, where the bath would have to be continued for weeks) as with pure dry heat. This *fact* is demonstrated by the Hot Springs of Arkansas. No one is benefited there who has weak and diseased lungs, but on the contrary, are made worse and are sent away. While in the Hot Air of the Turkish Bath, they are always relieved, (even in hopeless cases) and where there is simply functional derangement they invariably get well if they give it proper attention.

Women and the Bath.

Roman and Grecian ladies, famous for their beauty centuries ago, resorted constantly to the heated bath, knowing from experience its effect alike upon the beauty and upon the health, and centuries later, women noted for their wonderful charms even in old age. Ninon de l'Enclos and others, resorted to the bath as often as did the ancient beauties. They were enamored of it, knowing that so far as human charms could be increased and retained, the bath purifying constantly the system afforded the means. To-day, with the improvements made possible in the application of the bath by modern inventions, it is remarkable that the number of ladies who avail themselves of it is not far greater than in the past. The Turkish Bath is a more perfect thing—more completely adapted to enjoyment in taking it, and to promote health and beauty in its effects, than any bath available to the famous women of history. Yet now, instead of all, but the wiser of the ladies resort to it regularly.

The idea of womanly beauty without the accompanying idea of absolute bodily cleanliness and purity, is an impossible thing. Yet there are belles who forget the fact. It is a shocking thing to say, but there are women fair enough of feature and form, dressed richly, and graceful enough of carriage, who lack the greatest charm of all, unconscious of its very existence. The novelists and poets say, and it is an actual physical fact, that from the perfect cleanly body exhales a faint perfume, distinguishable to the senses It would be well were all women to remember this. There is no perfume exhaled from the form of the woman who never takes the bath.

Nature makes no distinctions, and the more beautiful of women have a skin which, while it may be originally whiter and softer, is as full of minute pores as is that of the coarsest men, and these minute pores, gradually filling, cannot be cleansed by the ordinary bath, and once clogged with impurities, produce sallowness, loss of perfect beauty of complexion, and what almost resembles disease. Even more susceptible than man is woman to this influence, which, particularly in the great cities where the air is loaded with impurities, is a constant thing. Whiteness and softness of skin and freshness of countenance, are the direct result of perfect care of the body; and as the dust and dirt of cities are artificial evils for which nature has not provided a remedy, so the Turkish Bath is an artificial means of counteracting these evils. It is the greatest of tonics, the best of cosmetics.

Ladies who have taken the Turkish Baths regularly need not be told all this. It is but a simple statement of a physical and medical fact for the benefit of those who have not yet learned the secret. It is not to be presumed that ladies who are enjoying the benefit of the Bath will keep from their friends the knowledge of what is the greatest of all preservatives of health and beauty; but they would, perhaps, be justified in doing so, since it is the natural desire of one woman to be fairer than another, and since they have at least a right to be silent on a delicate subject.

Of the value of the Turkish Bath in cases of weakness or disease of the class to which women alone are liable, much has been written and said, and the knowledge ought to be general. In this brief article it is but intended to call attention to those benefits of the Bath which are certain in every case, and which every Lady is seeking.   S. W.

The Value of the Turkish Bath to Business Men

Cannot be estimated in dollars and cents, as it is practically invaluable to them. None know better than the merchant, the book-keeper or the clerk that a dull, languid, lazy feeling is not alone prejudicial to their business interests, but is unpleasantly detrimental to health. The merchant, confined night and day by the laborious duties of his business, is mentally over-worked, and the main organs of life's citadel become paralyzed in their efforts to perform the functions imposed upon them by the laws of nature. The book-keeper, kept from morning until night at the desk, is restricted from all exercise, and he, too, becomes an easy, though unwilling victim to the fatal maladies that overtake those of sedentary habits. The clerk usually has no regular hours for meals, and is compelled to take a bite here and there, is exposed to draughts and colds, and generally becomes a confirmed dyspeptic, sickly, and of a melancholy nature. We here write of three distinctive classes of business men because they are the three most generally found suffering from various ills which do not for years incapacitate them entirely from work, but which finally become fatal in their effects. What is the remedy? asks one. What shall I do to be cured? asks another. Thank God, the intelligence and common sense of the ancients has been investigated and confirmed by the present age, and the Turkish Baths in their purity, simplicity and efficiency are recommended by all who have tested them as the most salient, powerful and effective cure for the ailments mentioned above. They are unfailing in their remedial action when properly used, and have done more towards benefiting the business men of St. Louis than all other remedies combined. Our bankers, lawyers, physicians, merchants, and others, all bear testimony to their wonderful effects on the system Not alone is the diseased body cleansed and purged of the seeds of disease, but in addition thereto the organs that sustain and regulate life, are restored to their pristine vigor and regularity. No man knows what it is to be clean until he has enjoyed the felicitous delights of the Turkish Baths, and no individual has tasted the cup of luxury unless he has revelled in this supremest of luxuries Why be ill, moping about and miserable, when the Turkish Bath will instil new life and new vigor?

DRUG DISEASES.

It is a fact on which the public cannot too seriously ponder, that, by the remorseless pursuit of their practices, drug doctors have succeeded in creating a multitude of new diseases, which they have themselves christened; principally, by the names of the different drugs, that are instrumental in causing them. It is an undisputed fact, that drugs, which are habitually and freely prescribed in ordinary cases of illness, are the causes of a multitude of the most serious diseases which among the profession are known as drug disease. I am certain, says Dr. E. Johnson, "*I speak the literal truth, the simple, the unexaggerated truth, when I assert that thousands—not hundreds—but thousands of human beings are killed every year, alone by drug medication.*"

There is nothing very novel in this practice, however, but let us look at the matter in detail.

Dr. Pereira, one of the most eminent authorities on "Materia Medica," and held in high estimation by the drug school—says of alkalies, which are in constant use, as *potash, soda, ammonia, magnesia*, that "by continued use they give rise to increased activity of the different secreting organs and of the absorbing vessels and glands; effects which are analogus to those caused by mercury. After some time, the digestive functions *becomes disordered, the appetite fails, the blood becomes thin and darker colored, and loses its power of spontaneous coagulation when drawn from the body*; the whole system, and more particularly the *digestive organs, become enfeebled, and a state precisely similar to that of scurvy is brought on.''*

The disease thus produced is called *alkaline scurvy*. Yet the treatment of rheumatic fever by alkalies is the popular thing.

Arsenic in the most minute doses, (Allopathic doses) produces a disease which the same authority, says—medical practitioners, *occasionally mistake for English cholera!*—or, infantile remittent, otherwise *gastric fever.''*

And he adds, the " mistake is *sometimes* attended with consequences equally *fatal to the patient* and the reputation of the physician.''

This pleasant disease figures in medical nosology as *Febris Arsenicalis.* Then there is another disease the same poison gives rise to, which is distinguished as *Arsenical Cephatitis*, from the fact that there is great inflammation of the head and face. The glands of the jaw and face become enlarged, as in a case Dr. Pereira quotes from a French authority, (Desgranges), " giddiness, fainting, burning sensation at the pit of the stomach, occasional vomiting, heat in micturation, constipation, trembling 'of the limbs, and delirium were also present.''

Iodine is a drug most freely prescribed in its simple or uncombined state, in tinctures, or as it exists in many preparations, and the disease to which its use gives rise, is called *Iodism*. According to Dr. Pereira, it is *a very dangerous medicine* for any one to take who is "disposed to dyspepsia," that is, "indigestion."

Dr. Thompson, Professor of Materia Medica in the London University, says of iodine, "Its primary influence is exerted upon the stomach, a fact which has been fully ascertained by the appearance observed on that organ in persons *who have been poisoned by it.*" And he adds, "Like other medicines, it *accumulates in the system*, and, therefore, the continued employment of it even in small doses, has occasionally(?) *proved fatal.*"

Mercury has long been regarded by the profession as the king, or queen bee, of medicine—a sovereign drug, under whatever gender, and it has been called, "the physician's sheet anchor." It is held to be a *sheet anchor* in fever, says Professor B. F. Barker, of New York Medical College. But it is an anchor *that moors your patient to the grave.* By its use alone hundreds upon hundreds of thousands have been slaughtered, and must necessarily continue to be slaughtered as long as its use is persevered in, while thousands upon thousands who, from one cause or other, it did not kill outright, have been disfigured and tormented for life by its disastrous effects on their system. The preparations in which this deadly poison consitutes the staple ingredient are very numerous, but that most commonly administered is known as *calomel*, or the chloride of mercury. It matters not, however, in powder or pill, combined or sublimated, it destroys life rapidly, or by protracted agony, according as it is administered, while it has the peculiar merit of being the prolific parent of a number of *new diseases*, the very mention, or rather the enumeration of which, it is horrible to contemplate. To make my point good, and to clinch the nail right here, I quote from the *Allopathic Text-Books* a few of the many new diseases *caused* by the use of mercury, (in its different combinations) which the world never would have been cursed with—if *medical science* had not introduced mercury as a *curative agent in disease.*

1. *Febris Erethica Nel Salivosa*—Inflammatory, or salivary fever.

2. *Erethismus Mercurialis*—A fever characterized by prostration and depression. The action of the heart will sometimes cease instantaneously, and death ensue.

3. *Mercurial Enteritis*—Mercurial inflammation of the bowels.

4. *Eczema Mercuriale*—Mercurial skin disease.

5. *Mercurial Cachexia*—Characterized by irritable circulation, external pallor, and emaciation; hectic fever, and almost invariably terminating in phthisis (consumption.)

6. *Tremor Mercurialis.*

7. *Mercurial Stomatitis*—A disease that ensues when salivation has been designedly effected, *but cannot be subdued.* De Pereira states: "A few grains of blue pill administered for a liver complaint, brought it on in a female, and in another instance that of a child four years old. The latter was produced by a few grains of calomel!"

8. *Diarrhœa Mercurialis*—Mercurial purging, or mercurial disease of the pancreas.

9. *Urorrhea Mercurialis*—A kind of mercurial diabetis, or rather diuresis

10. *Hidrosis Mercurialis*—Mercurial sweats.

11. *Miliaria Mercurialis*—A form of skin disease.

12. *Angina Mercurialis*—A mercurial inflammation and sloughing of the gullet.

13. *Neuralgia Mercurialis*—Induced by mercury.

14. *Paralysis Mercurialis*—Same cause.

15. *Apoplexia Mercurialis*—Use of Mercury.

16. *Amaurosis Mercurialis*—Dimness of sight, or total blindness.

And so on to the end of the chapter; but the above named are sufficient to convince all but *idiots* that mercury is not a healing balm, *but the devil's own drug*; and as I have remarked above, if drug practitioners had never dosed their victims with mercury, the above diseases, with scores of others I could name, would never have been known. Dr Thompson, who is often quoted as high authority in *Materia Medica* says: "Mercurial Preparations, whether chlorides, cyanides, or iodides, are decomposed, and the mercury, in a metallic form, is either thrown out of the body by the *skin or lungs*, or under *certain circumstances is deposited in the glands or bones*." Because the tendency of mercury is to produce fatal diseases. He says, "On this account *mercurials should be introduced into the system gradually, and the mildest forms of the preparations first employed*." A slow death, the professor of *Materia Medica* thinks, preferable to a rapid one! !

Under the circumstances, it seems to me a person

with any common sense would ask, " Why introduce it into the system at all in any shape or form? But no, it is said, we must not ask questions ; we employ a physician, and if he don't know, who should?

What is this world coming to if we are to doubt our family physician, who is educated, made drugs his study, etc., etc. That is what's the matter. He has made *Materia Medica* his study, instead of Physiology and the laws of health. How to cure the sick, instead of how to keep them well. They take the bull by the tail (to use a homely phrase,) instead of by the horns, and until medical schools change their methods com pletely, the drug doctors are not the ones to take charge of the individual sick, or look after the sanitary interests of the community.

THE TURKISH BATH.

A few weeks ago an event occurred which offered occasion for writing the history of the Turkish Bath in St. Louis, and one of our prominent morning papers improved the opportunity; unfortunately, however, the information imparted in the historical sketch then given was, aside of its incompleteness, so inaccurate as to confound the entire article. With an anticipation of the importance which the Bath must, ere long, obtain as a remedial agent for all diseases as well also as a preventive against the worst ills peculiar to our climate, it becomes our duty to correct the errors of that sketch, and thereby place upon the records the true history of the introduction and establishment of the Turkish Bath in our city.

In the fall of 1868, Judge Thomas T. Gantt, being impressed with the invaluable uses of the bath, opened a correspondence with Dr. Geo. F. Adams, at the time proprietor of two Turkish Bath establishments in Boston, with the view of obtaining his opinion and assistance in the construction of similar bath-rooms in St. Louis. During the correspondence several prominent St. Louis gentlemen visited Dr. Adams' institutions in

Boston, and became so infatuated with the luxury and effects of the bath, that they at once joined with Judge Gantt in urging Dr. Adams to come to St. Louis and see what could be done towards establishing a bath here. Some of Judge Gantt's friends, however, subsequently became lukewarm towards the enterprise, but he continued his best endeavors, and finally succeeded in raising $18,000, although $40,000 was the sum fixed upon. Dr. Adams came to St. Louis, and, after considering the proposition, he was authorized to return to Boston and procure the plans and specifications. This being done, Dr. Adams arrived in St. Louis January 15th, 1869, but found that little had been done towards perfecting arrangements during his absence. His return, however, infused new life in the enterprise and the work of securing additional funds to carry out the project properly was begun again by Judge Gantt, who gave a public lecture on the subject in Polytechnic Hall, which was largely attended. Shortly after the lecture an association was formed and a charter obtained from the State for the incorporation of the Turkish Bath Company in St. Louis. Among the names of the organizers were T. T. Gantt, C. T. Burns, Joseph O'Neil, and several more of our best citizens.

Thus far the friends of the bath felt confident of its early establishment, but now another barrier interposed itself and prevented the success of the enterprise thus seemingly auspiciously inaugurated. The balance of the necessary funds could not be raised, and finally it was declared the time was not ripe for the investment of so much money in a new thing.

In the February following, Mr. Robinson, (lately deceased) who was at that time proprietor of a large barber shop, at No. 410 Market Street, approached Dr. Adams and engaged him to superintend the building of a small Turkish Bath as an auxiliary to his barber shop. Accordingly, the Doctor made the plans, furnished drawings for the couches and plumbing, heating flues, ventilation, and all the work was done under his direction. The work occupied only a few weeks, and, when the bath was ready for use, the Doctor furnished Mr. Robinson with the necessary instructions for giving the baths properly; taught the attendants to shampoo, and thus engaged for several weeks, gave Mr. Robinson the experience for conducting the institution satisfactorily.

Dr. Adams, having disposed of his Boston establishments, determined to try the experiment suggested by Judge Gantt, and when, in the following spring, the corporate body abandoned the enterprise entirely, the Doctor built a bath at No. 1603 Washington Avenue, which was opened to the public October 8th, 1869, and for three years proved a financial success. The increase of patronage finally exceeded the capacity of the institution and the Doctor was induced, in 1872, to build another and larger bath at No. 311 North Seventh Street. This last establishment was completed and opened June 20th, 1873. The Doctor continued to run the Washington Avenue bath, but reserved it for ladies exclusively. This venture, however, proved a failure, the cause being found in various reasons not necessary to particularize in this connection. The Doctor then closed his Washington Avenue branch and confined his attention to his main bath on Seventh street, devoting three mornings of each week to ladies, the patronage from whom is now so great that to accommodate them properly more time is being asked. It is no more than proper to state here that Dr. Adams is one of the oldest and best experienced Turkish Bath proprietors in this country, and his bath rooms at 311 North Seventh Street, being built without regard to cost, is the most complete institution of the kind west of New York city.

The true history of the Turkish Bath in St. Louis ascribes to Judge T. T. Gantt the honor of first bringing the virtues of the bath before our citizens, and to Dr. Geo. F. Adams the credit for building the first bath room, and giving it a firm footing in the estimation of St. Louisians.

Better Than · Milk.

In the time of "the Directory," in France,
  Skins fair and soft as silk
Were counted but as charms of circumstance;
  They said: "She's bathed in milk."
When speaking of some famous reigning belle,
  Some court of beauty's queen,
Of whom e'en yet, the poets love to tell
  Whose portrait yet is seen.
Times change, yet woman's beauty is the same,
  And to assure her reign
By proper means. as sought the storied dame,
  Will haughtiest woman deign;
But. wiser than her sister of that day,
  The present beauty hath
Learned to enhance her charms, a surer way—
  She takes the Turkish Bath.

Our Own Experience.

Doctor Herberden once said, in "Politics and Morality" : "*Experience* may be called the the teacher of fools, but in the study of *nature, there is no other guide to true knowledge.*" This is conclusive, however, only in one point—that the most extensive practice, when based on erroneous principles, can never become natural and truthful, nor lead to desirable results ; and also, that Experience, no matter how enlarged and prolonged—operating on ill-trained, ill-educated minds warped by prejudice, like seed sown on a desert of sand, is never destined to take root and fructify.

Yet Experience, wisely employed, is invaluable to a medical practitioner capable of following and profiting by its unerring teachings. It stands in opposition to the speculative theories and fanciful systems of physic which, propagated by schools, has inflicted incalculable misery on mankind, and which are now followed as keenly as ever.

If a physician is asked for a reason for giving a certain drug in such and such a disease, his answer invariably is : "*My experience teaches* me that it is useful in such cases." Nothing can be more convenient than this answer. But, then, if you walk right straight from physician No 1 to physician No. 2, he will, in nine cases out of ten, give you a drug whose *nature* and *effects* are as different from that prescribed by No. 1 physician as any two things can well be. Yet, if you inquire of No. 2 why he orders for your case the particular drug or drugs he prescribes, he will give you the same answer as the first. He will tell you that *experience* has satisfied him that the drug he has ordered for you is useful in such cases. At this rate *remedies for diseases must be as plentiful as blackberries.* But what possible reliance can be placed upon this kind of experience of any one out of twenty men, when it is found that the experience of each of the twenty is contradicted by the experience of all the others? Every man prescribes according to his own experience.

The truth is, that what they call experience is *mere accident. But* my experiences that I propose to give in this article are not *accidental* or *jumped at*, but a *positive* and *real* experience. " The study of nature is the only guide to knowledge " in matters appertaining to the laws of life and health.

For thirteen years and more I have devoted all my time, all my energies, (and what little skill I may have attained in a practice of more than thirty years), to the principles and the merits of the " Hot-Air Bath " as a remedial agent. Seconded earnestly and faithfully by my wife—partly from the fact that it gave me courage and pleasure, and partly from the satisfaction manifested by her patrons, who visited the Bath for its novel and new way of bathing, as well as those who came for its remedial effects—we have worked together earnestly and unremittingly; and although the balance on the Ledger is on the wrong side, yet we have the satisfaction of knowing that hundreds of thousands have enjoyed the great luxury, and that thousands of ladies and gentlemen have been restored to perfect health through the instrumentality of the Bath. Though sacrifices (both financial and social) have been made, yet we feel well repaid in the thought that, some time in the far future, our *almost gratuitous* labors will be appreciated by a wiser and more enlightened generation.

I feel some reluctance in speaking of my experience, in consequence of the utter unreliability of *medical experience* as portrayed above. Still, my experience is a new one; and as I have no favors to ask of any one, no opponents to punish, and no possible object in view but to relate it, honestly and truthfully, I must allow my readers to draw their own conclusions.

My experience leads me to believe that ninety-nine out of one hundred bathers who use the Bath for cleanliness and for sanitary purposes, are delighted with it, and recommend it. In chronic cases of disease all are benefited, and where there is no organic disease they invariably get well, if they give it proper time and attention. My experience leads me to believe that many organic diseases have been cured through the instrumentality of the Hot-Air Bath. I will explain, and give reasons for the faith that is in me. I have had in my charge many cases of Bright's Disease of the kidneys. The patients stated to me that for months they had been under treatment for this disease; that they had had consultations with the ablest medical men of this city, and that their decision was Bright's Disease. Indeed, in two cases I saw and conversed with their family physicians; they informed me that their cases were hopeless, but remarked that if the patients could be made to sweat their lives might be prolonged, but that they never could get well.

One of those patients visited the Bath sixty-three days in succession. So feeble was he at first that he was brought in a carriage the first twenty days. His health improved steadily—his weight was reduced from 140 pounds to 105, often losing from 4 to $5\frac{1}{2}$ pounds each Bath. In less than four months he was perfectly well, and has remained so, now eight years. I need not say that he still continues his weekly Bath, and that he credits the Bath for his physical salvation. I have had many such cases come under my observation, and nearly all have recovered. Hundreds of cases of kidney diseases, in their different phases, have recovered while using the Bath. If the patient is entirely under my care I invariably advise him to let drugs alone; and, by the way, I here declare that patients who let drugs entirely alone, improve faster than those who dose while taking a course of Baths.

Chronic Diarrhœa, every one knows, (especially physicians) how troublesome and vexatious such cases are to treat by drugs—or rather in the regular way, yields to the soothing influence of the "Hot Air Bath." One case in point. Some two or three years since a gentleman from Whitehall, Ill., age, past sixty, stated his case thus-wise: I have been out of health for more than six years; have suffered from chronic diarrhœa most of the time; have employed the best doctors in this city and country; have been to all the springs I know of, of any note; have spent the last winter in Georgia, and am to-day, worse than I was

when I went South in the fall, etc., etc.; and now I
want to try the bath as a dernier resort, but I have no
hope. He commenced taking the baths that day,
April 10th. He continued them for two or three
weeks; was much improved; he had faith. He sent
for his wife. Rented a small house in the suburbs;
continued the baths until October, when he returned
home in perfect health, and has remained so up to the
present time. Here was a case of ulceration of the
bowels, *organic disease* his former physicians pronounced it, and no possible chance for his recovery.
Many similar cases have been treated in the same
way—without drugs—with the same results. Chronic
bronchitis—hopelessly sick to all appearance, has
been successfully treated in the "Hot Air Bath."
One case only, I propose to refer to. One of our
most prominent insurance men had been under treatment for months by one of our eminent physicians in
the city, treated of course, "secundum artem," but
he grew worse, and that continually. Dr. —— advised him to visit Denver, and gave him a letter of
introduction to a physician of that city—the patient
continued to grow worse under the same kind of
treatment he had at home, and finally he became dis-
gusted with drug medication and quit it, and commenced a course of "Hot Air Baths" in Denver. To
use his own words, "it worked like a charm. I be-
gan to breathe through my skin, but my cough was
still terrific. But I persevered, was much improved
in a few weeks, and returned as far as Kansas City.
Continued the baths for six weeks—and here I am—
and I want to continue the good work with you if it
takes a year." This gentleman was a perfect wreck

physically. Skin and bones, so to speak. He continued to improve and is now well. Weighing seventy pounds more than when he went to the mountains.

These few chronic cases mentioned, are simply to show what a *splendid physician nature* is, when trusted, and when not interfered with by those who actually boast of doing their work. *Curing disease, as they call it,* better than the Creator. Hundreds of chronic cases are treated monthly. All are benefited.

Acute diseases are controlled by the bath. I might say truthfully, in a marvelous way, as well as prevented.

As a sanitary measure, my experience leads me to say that I have an abiding faith that the Turkish Bath bather will be almost, if not altogether, exempt from infectious diseases, and I do not over estimate my faith in saying so

My first years experience in Saint Louis fortified my belief in the above statement. Small pox was raging as an epidemic. A tenement house standing next door to my bath and residence, contained seven families, five of these families had more or less cases of the disease. Servants were wild with fright, and every body about the house was alarmed. I was urged repeatedly to be vaccinated. Also to have my son and another boy living with us. I finally consented to have the boys attended to—but I insisted also that they should take the hot air bath every day, as they and all the rest of the family had been doing for several weeks. The boys were vaccinated three times in as many weeks, but it did not take. I had them both vaccinated the fourth time, and omitted the bath. They both had what is called *good arms*. It is also a fact, (and I presume there are scores who will certify to what I am about to say) every gentleman, every one who had been vaccinated, and to all appearance was going to take, the slight inflammatory appearance disappeared and the scab dried and fell off. From these facts physicians and others can draw their own conclusions.

I feel that they are worthy of more than a passing notice.

Local inflammation, such as inflamed eyes, carbuncles, boils, inflamed and swollen glands, are more readily relieved with one bath of an hours' duration, than could possibly be achieved by local applications in a day, if at all. I have seen a little girl with granulated eye-lids, for two years and more suffering (blind in one eye, and she could not bear day-light with the other,) recover her sight—granulations completely absorbed, general health completely restored, by simply attending the bath. No medicines were given, no local applications, except soft, linen cloths wet in warm water while bathing, and the same used on going to bed at night. This was accomplished in about six months' time, under the most unfavorable circumstances. The girl had been in the hands of the most excellent oculists in this city for more than two years.

Chorea, in its most violent and destructive forms, has been permanently cured by the bath. *Insomnia* is always cured by the bath. In many instances I have known bathers to go to sleep immediately after coming into the cooling room from the bath—in some instances where the patient had not been able to sleep for weeks, everything in the shape of anodynes having failed.

All zymotic diseases are completely controlled by the judicious application of the bath.

This kind of experience is so satisfactory to me that I am anxious to have all physicians avail themselves of this same knowledge that passeth all understanding. But I have already expatiated too much upon my experience, though it could be extended to an unlimited extent, but will close by saying that during thirteen years and more, not an accident of any moment has occurred, although patrons from three years old to eighty-five, have visited us. Sick and feeble invalids, the athlete, men and women of sedentary habits, the robust and the healthy, all join in one accord to praise the inestimable value of the Turkish Bath in health, as well as in disease. One hundred and forty odd thousand names registered in our books join in this universal cry. Compare my experience with the experience discussed in the first part of this article. But comparisons are————etc., etc.

Exercise and Cleanliness.

When we think of it, most of the forms of medical treatment consist in the administration of *exercise*. This exercise may be internal or external in its application, local or general, organic or constitutional. What men need when they are sick is some mode of exercise. Sickness implies that there is some arrest of function, some sluggishness of circulation, some congestion or want of equalization in the system, which exercise, properly applied, might remedy. One man takes calomel and gives his liver a somersault; another takes salts, and puts his stomach and intestines in a state of tribulation: one takes digitalis and stimulates the heart; another, with quinine, chords up the nervous system.

If we step outside the province of drugs, we have the Swedish mountain cure, the health lift, light gymnastics, manipulations, electricity, walking, riding. And all these may serve an admirable purpose, each in its own way. But not one of these combines so many hygienic qualities as the Turkish Bath. Indeed, we are almost tempted to ask what health-giving agency is wanting in this excellent device and remedy, while in several respects it is unapproachable in its salutary effects.

The weak patient may not be able to take riding so as to make it remedial; or the man exhausted by busi-

ness cannot further spare his vitality to take a walk.
He needs exercise, no doubt. He may have been on
his feet all day, at the counter, or sitting at his desk,
busy at his books. With little energy left for active
exertion—with possibly, also, a little pulmonary weakness, a little indigestion, a slight headache, a touch of
rheumatism, and some signs of biliousness, he is unfitted to take active exercise. He must have passive
exercise, i. e., he must have treatment in some shape.
He may try some drug or tonic; he may try electric
shocks or the health-lift; he may pack in cold water or
eat bran bread, but he will frequently find that after
trying all, the Turkish Bath is the one remedy that
meets his case. It is the best passive exercise known.

In the first place, this Bath is exactly suited to the
weak or tired man, disordered in his nerves and jaded
with care. He has only to submit, Nothing is required
of him. The heat is grateful and soothing. He lies
down to absolute quiet for a while, then he is manipu-
lated by the hand of the shampooer in every part of the
body, until every muscle is touched and toned with the
animal magnetism of the operator. Every internal
organ feels the gentle effect of the manipulating and
kneading process, while the skin glows with the imparted activity and health. The liver is relieved by this
cleansing of the pores, the circulation equalized, the
pulse tempered, the nerves quieted.

How few persons realize the importance of attention
to the state of the pores of the skin. Half the diseases of this sooty, dusty city would be relieved or
averted if the skin were kept in good condition.
Then every miasmatic climate doubles the difficulty

and the danger. The cutaneous perspiration (or "transpiration," as Dr. Carpenter calls it), sensible and insensible, is probably twice as great in a man living in the Mississippi Valley, as in one living in Colorado or in New England. Now, if the pores are choked with biliary deposits—if the capillaries are paralyzed with the poison of jaundice and malaria, (which ordinary bathing is often utterly ineffective to remove)—I confess I know no remedy like the Turkish Bath. Nor has a man any safety or immunity from disease while the skin is in this sluggish and unwholesome condition. The intimate relation which the cutaneous excretion bears to bilious, urinary and kidney diseases is known to all physiologists. Experiments upon the lower animals by Drs. Foreault and Becquerel, show that the suppression of perspiration by covering the skin with varnish, glue or suet, rapidly lowers the temperature, prevents the arterialization of the blood, tends to congestion of the internal organs, causes albuminaria, and in time cutaneous asphyxia and death.

J. C. L.

MY FIRST BATH.

I had a cold. I had starved it and fed it, and cough *mixtured* it, and smothered it in flannel, but it still held on with the leech-like tenacity of an insurance agent or a poor relation. I tried the *regular* practice, wishing to be healed in a respectable, orthodox fashion. Then I ran after the "strange gods" of Homœopathy, Electropathy, Thompsoniansy, but I gained nothing, either in restored health or respectability of character. One man suggested "Whiskey and Rock Candy." I took the whisky and gave the candy to the baby. A mustard plaster was recommended. I made my spinal column externally resemble an overdone lobster, and feel like the back of Mazeppa after he had finished his celebrated bare-back act. I then swallowed three half pints of red-pepper tea, and felt as Mount Vesuvius must feel when the wind is the wrong way! Finally, somebody suggested a "cold pack." They wrapped me in a wet sheet, and I felt as if I had suddenly discovered the North Pole. Then they covered me to the chin in blankets, while I sweated in helpless anguish, shrouded and bandaged in woolen, like Lazarus in the Tomb; a singularly alert fly waltzed on the tip of my nose until I shrieked with the tickle. Then a friend said "try a Turkish Bath." Now, like most people who are densely ignorant about

the matter, I had very decided, and carefully matured
convictions upon this subject. I felt that the Turkish
Bath was the last expiring gasp of the Spanish inquisi-
sition, or an imperfect substitute for that place which
Mr. Beecher calls obsolete. I had been told and
implicitly believed that when a respectable, wealthy
old citizen had a son inclined to imitate the only
scriptural model that seems to be popular among the
sons of our first families—the Prodigal—he took him
to the Turkish Bath, as an awful warning against his
possible future.

I said I would consult the doctors; so I did. Their
testimony against the bath was unanimous. They had
never seen it in operation. Had always steadily
refused to listen to the intelligent testimony of any one
who had. Still they argued like this: If the bath
was a good thing, why did they not use it? They did
not use it, *ergo*, etc., etc. One doctor described the process as analogous to the steaming of a Murphy potato.
Another thought it was a kind of human *laundry*, in
which the body was possibly run through a patent cog-
wheel clothes wringer. They all believed, in general
terms, that it was another "section of the *ragged edge*
of the day of judgment," and only needed a skillful
imitation of the shrieking of the damned to make the
illusion complete. The bath might clean me, it could
never cure me. And they felt like the charity body
in relation to the alphabet. They did not believe it
paid to go through so much to gain so little. Still I
did not get better, and in fear and trembling I went to
the Bath. I made my will previous to the visit, and
took a more than ordinarily affectionate leave of my
household—was careful to obtain legal advice respect-

ing the validity of my life insurance claim, in case I perished under the heroic treatment. Then I came, I saw, I *was* conquered. Prejudice rolled away from my mind, as the porous accumulations of years rolled from my frame. I discovered then what I had long suspected, viz., that St. Louis dust really penetrates the immortal soul, and will in time clog the delicate operation of the conscience. Under the dry heat my lightened spirit cast off its load of undeveloped sin, and I came back to mankind morally rejuvenated. My inner nature re-assumed its child-like and pristine purity. I felt like a good Catholic coming from confession It was as if I had been only *Baptized* by every ex denomination in town. I was neither baked, boiled, smothered nor steamed. I fell into a gentle slumber, under the serene influence of 150 degrees in the shade. I left that place a converted man. Now, when I have a cold, a head-ache, a back-ache, an *all-over-ache*, when I am tired and blue, and feel as if life was an investment that did not pay 1 per cent., I go to the "Bath," and the clouds roll away, and I feel as happy as a gum-chewing school girl with her first trail.   NEMO.

A Little Nonsense Now and Then, Etc.

LABOR NOT LOST; Or, All's Well that Ends Well.

DRAMATIS PERSONÆ.

HAMLET Prince of Denmark.	HAL Prince of Wales.	
MACBETH King of Scotland.	BRUTUS A Patriot.	
SIR JOHN FALSTAFF Knight.	ROMEO A Sick Lover.	

Clerks, Attendants, Turks.

SCENE I.—311 *North Seventh St. at Noon. Enter* HAL.

HAL. And that fat-witted rogue comes hither
I'll play him such a trick that Doll, his leman,
Shan't know his face when next he goes her way.

Enter FALSTAFF.

FAL. A plague on this gout, say I;
This drinking of old sack has spoiled my waist,
Made gross this erst slight figure, and undone
The goodliest master piece of human flesh
That ever came from Mother Nature's mould.
Hal, you here?

HAL. How now, fat knave; why lookest thou so sour?

FAL. I'm sorely tried, Hal, and surely do I feel
That my good life is drawing to a close.
Commend me to some leech whose skill shall make
Your valiant Falstaff a sound man again.

HAL. 'Tis just my humor, Jack; go seek this place,
'Twill ease thy pains, make fair thy bloated face.
                    [*Hands* FALSTAFF *a slip of paper. Exit.*]

FALSTAFF [*reading*] The Bath.
Hot air, tis curious; still I go
To make this cast for happiness or woe.   [*Exit.*]

Enter HAMLET, HAL *following him unperceivea.*

HAMLET.   To be or not to be—that is the question
Whether 'tis nobler in the mind to suffer
The Slings—Good Day, Prince Harry.

HAL.   Now faith, sweet Hamlet, you look not well;
Thy clothes hang loose about thee; and thine eye
Wears not that joysome glance I've marked of yore,
When we were boys together.
Art in love, good Hamlet?

HAMLET.   Even so, fair Prince.

HAL.   Woulds't find thyself in better frame of mind.
Dispel the shadows that oppress thy soul,
And be once more a merry, Danish Prince.

HAMLET.   Marry would I.

HAL.   This missive take.
Obey, and 'ere the morrow's sun has dawned
Hamlet shall be himself again.
[*Reads*] Seek ye the Bath.
Ay, kind friend, I will;
And should it ease this malady of brain
Hamlet, indeed, will be himself again.

SCENE II.—*The Office of the Turkish Bath.   Cierk Seated at desk*

Enter FALSTAFF.

FAL.   Good master clerk, my Prince has bid me here
To test the powers of this woudrous Bath.

CLERK.   Welcome, Sir John.   Your hat and sword,
And now one dollar and a quarter—the fee.

FAL.   Out, Knave, my knightly word;
Will that suffice?

CLERK.   Not here, sir John; hard cash, an' please you, sir.

FAL.   A murrain on thee.   Here's the coin;
But if thy bath does not my gout assuage
I'll cudgel thee.   Come, lead me in.

Enter HAMLET, MACBETH *and* HAL.

MAC.   Sleep, I'll sleep no more.
Hallo, Prince Henry, and our Hamlet, too.

HAMLET.   What seeks the great Thane here?

MAC.   Repose, young Prince; for mind and body rest.

HAL.   Thou hast chosen well, oh, Thane;
Enter, and bid a long farewell to pain.
[*All enter bath, followed by Attendants.*

SCENE III.—*Interior of the Bath.* HAMLET, FALSTAFF, MACBETH, and HAL *perspiring.*

FAL. Now, beshrew me, Hal, if ever on Gadshill
My lard did ooze so freely as this hour.
Nay, mark it wet the floor
With the best juices of a saintly man.

Enter ROMEO.

ROMEO. Oh, good attendant on this stricken heart
Let your shampooing hand fall tenderly.
So, so even now I feel a great relief.
Your touch, kind sir, so gentle and so bland.
Reminds me of the gentle Juliet's hand.
MAC. What soothing balm is here!
Conscience grows easy, and the eating cares
Of grim misdeeds fall one by one away.
Methinks were Banquo's ghost to rise up here
With tranquil mind I'd bid the shade good cheer.

Enter BRUTUS.

BRUTUS. You gentlemanly sir has led me hither
And told me that the grief I carry with me
For Caesar's death would in this peaceful place
Soon disappear.
FAL. Ho! Roman friend, hast thou the gout?
Or have the doctors made thee sick, or doth
Great Caesar's death weigh heavy on thy mind?
BRUTUS. Not all remorse, Sir John.
'Tis mixed with rheumatism which I caught
On the Campagna several months ago.
HAL. Then rest thee here, noble Brutus.
Here shalt thou be made hale to slay
A dozen Caesars for thy country's good.

[*All adjourn to the Shampooing Room.*]

SCENE IV.—*The office of the Bath.* Clerk reckoning FALSTAFF's *account for drinks and cigars.*

Enter ROMEO, MACBETH, HAL. FALSTAFF, BRUTUS, *and* HAMLET.

HAL. Now, sirs, that ye have bathed, I bid ye tell
If this good bath hath eased your several pains.

FAL. Hamlet, thou art a brick.
This belly, which, like a Saratoga trunk,
I carried in, has shrunk away and left
The goodliest knight in all this Christian land,
Honest Jack Falstaff, light, and brave, and gay.
I swear I'll come here every second day.

HAL. And you, Macbeth?

MAC. The change is marvelous;
My peace of mind restored,
My frame is sound, eased is my aching brain;
And Birnam Wood may come to Dunsinane
A thousand times before it scares this Thane.

ROMEO. I'll think of naught but Juliet.
Away with Friar Laurence's gloomy fears,
I'll to my Juliet fly and tell her all
This process for her Romeo has achieved.
I'm changed so much I'm sure to be believed.

HAMLET. How now, my friends, it seems to me you wear
A different visage each since last I saw
Your faces underneath the bounteous showers.

HAL. How feels the gentle Prince?

HAMLET. Beyond all telling, Harry.
Even that old Polonius could not now
Disturb the even current of my thoughts.
I'll go and hug Ophelia.

BRUTUS *enters humming the " Sweet By and By."*

BRUTUS. Now, by Diana's temple, I could slay
Old Caesar o'er again and never feel
That aught but good lay in the patient steel.

ATTENDANT. Sir John, your coat.

FAL. Thanks, knave, a warm garment, faith.

HAL. Drop that, Jack, 'tis mine. Now, gentlemen,
When cares of mind, or any of those ills
That flesh is heir to, weigh your spirits down.
Leave here the cross and bear away the crown
Of joyous health. Farewell, we'll meet again
Within this sanctuary from human pain. .

[CURTAIN.]

—[*From San Francisco Hammam.*

PERSONAL AND GENERAL.

If the readers of this work think or believe that I have over-estimated the evils of drug treatment, or that I have been uncharitable towards the old school Profession (in other words, the Regulars) all will please bear in mind that I have, in every instance, quoted the sayings and writings of the best writers, the highest authorities, and as profound scholars as have ever lived, and all are acknowledged as such in the Medical world—all of which are of the Allopathic school, or were. I have myself seen more human *suffering and misery caused directly from the drug treatment* than from all other causes combined, during a life of more than sixty years. I believe, also, that I am not alone in such belief—that any honest Allopathic Physician who has been in practice forty years, or even less, will agree with me in many of my assertions, if not all.

To fortify myself still further in the above statements, I quote from *Boerhave*, (Med. Inst., page 401) : " If one comes to weigh without passion, the good done by a handful of *true sons of Æsculapius*, and the evils that the immense number of physicians have occasioned to the human race since the origin of that science until the present day, without doubt one would think that it would be more profitable that there had never been a physician in this world." *Stahl* estimated at seventy per cent the number of patients dying the fault of physicians. Speaking a little further about the allopathic therapeutics, he says: "I would wish that a bold hand would undertake to clean out that Augean stable. Very courageous is he who dares to study that science *so much crowded with errors.* Where the language is just as much *defensive* as the thought, and where everything is to be done over again, the principles just as well as the materials." *Gritanner pretends:* "That the darkness surrounding the practice of medicine is so thick that it is impossible for a ray of sunlight to penetrate into it, in order to enable anybody to direct its course." "Alas!" says he, "who will be able to discover the few good grains lost in the immense amount of chaff that physicians have accumulated during 4000 years." Dr. Borden cries: "Thirty years have I *guessed*, and I am tired of guessing."

Dr. Gilibert has given us a rule, "that the most learned physicians are the most dangerous, and that these are those that kill the greatest number of patients *because they doubt nothing.*"

Dr. Barthez, as celebrated a physician as Doctor Borden, emphatically declared that he did not believe in medical skill. "We are," he says, "blind men hitting with a stick at the disease, *or at the patient*—so much the better *for the patient if we strike the disease.*"

Dr. Bichat, the great anatomist, has said "that materia medica is of all sciences the one where is to be found the finest illustration of the oddities of the human mind; which I say is not a science; it is nothing else but an informal compound of incorrect ideas, of trifling observations, of illusory means, of fantastical formulas."

The learned physician, Kappart, says : " Medicine, poor science! Physicians, poor savants! Patients, poor victims!" And a little further on he says : " At least every twenty years the same school changes its system. Sometimes there are two or three systems in the same school ; in fact, among physicians from the same school, and having the same system, there are not four of them able to agree before a patient's bed."

Medical science is in a complete anarchy. That the profession is in a decline, and on the edge of an abyss. You have no medical body ; you live isolated in the enmity and contempt of one another ; the disfavor overruns yourselves ; from every part you are without resistance, as well as without power, and the least shock, long and boldly repeated, will finish and ruin you. I am free to confess that I have the most profound disgust for drug practice, and an honest contempt for the means often resorted to by many of the profession to gain a livelihood—

" Ways that are dark, and tricks that are vain."

The whole secret of the " Turkish Bath " over the sources and springs of life, consists in facilitating by natural means the process of renovation. *Liebig*, who is authority of the highest repute, has testified "by means of the Turkish Bath treatment *a change of matter* is effected in a greater degree in *six weeks*, than would happen in the *ordinary* course of nature in *three years*," a bold statement, but nevertheless I believe it

true, for my twelve years' experience in administering
the bath teaches me that the bath acts naturally, salub-
riously and promptly, with a marvelous and unerring
certainty that nothing else can equal, in facilitating the
renewal process of organic life.

It will thus be understood that to preserve health,
and to prevent disease, are the great sanitary ends to
be obtained by the judicious use of the Bath. As a
social institution it is one of the grandest luxuries one
can treat himself to. Briefly, *health is preserved* by
the instrumentality of the Bath, maintaining in vigorous action the vital organism of the skin, on which the
functions of circulation, nutrition and elimination so
largely depend.

Disease is prevented by hardening the body against
the effects of variations and vicissitudes of temperature, which is of incalculable advantage in a climate so
variable as ours ; and last, but not least, by imparting
power to resist miasmatic and zymotic influences, and
furthermore, by correcting, eradicating or keeping in
subjection inherited predisposition to disease. In this
way the Bath rises to the dignity of an unequalled sanitary institution, and the time is not far distant when it
will be so acknowledged by the profession.

————

If the inestimable value of the Turkish Bath were
known and fully understood—as a remedial agent in
disease—as a preventive in the thousand-and-one diseases the human family are liable to—if, I say, these
facts were known, St. Louis would boast of a dozen
first-class baths to-day instead of one. Our hospitals
and insane asylums, also, would be blessed with this

great *boon to* humanity, for such it would be to the
unfortunate ones, who, through misfortune or other
causes are obliged to resort to these charitable institutions. Not a physician in the land would dare, even
if from selfish motives or other disparaging reasons
they were inclined to do so, raise their voices against
it, for the whole community, rich and poor, would
silence their objections. The Boards of Health of every
city in the Union would insist upon the introduction of
the " Hot Air Bath " into every institution over which
they had control.

In all ages, past as well as present, there have been
minds so constituted and cultivated as to find in experience *a true source of knowledge*, but they are to be
counted as units in comparison with the millions of ill-
constituted, ill-cultivated minds that have only found
in experience a confirmation of their prejudices and
errors. Hence, to the great majority of medical practitioners, experience performs the same office, and with
precisely similar results in the authentication of erroneous preconceptions, as in the case of the Sultan—
described by Byron—who

> Saw, by his own eyes, the moon was round;
> Was, also, certain that the earth was square,
> Because he had journied fifty miles, and found
> No signs that it was circular anywhere.

An eminent and candid medical authority, Dr.
Frank, of London, once said: " *thousands are annu-
ally slaughtered in the quiet sick-room,*" and as the
Regulars make common cause, they say to the relatives
and friends of the victims immolated by their gross and

palpable blundering, that science and art had been skillfully employed to effect a cure, but that it was God's will—His time had come—and that is all that can be said about it.

Dr. Ramage, of London, placed the following remarkable opinion on record: "I fearlessly assert, that in most cases *the patient would be safer without a physician than with one.* I have seen enough of the mal-practice of my professional brethren to warrant the strong language I employ."

Dr. John Johnson, for many years editor of the *Medico Chirurgical Review*, gives his independent testimony thus: "I declare, as my conscientious conviction, founded on long experience and reflection, that if there was not a single physician, man-midwife, chemist, apothecary, druggist, nor drug on the face of the earth, there would be less sickness and less mortality than now prevails."

It should never be forgotten that the universe moves in obedience to laws so wise and good that they will never require to be amended, altered or revoked. It is the proper business of true science and philosophy to work in harmony with these laws. They have forever connected health with temperance and peace with virtue. For one I indulge the hope that science will fully unfold the mystery of our being and show the law of our progress written upon all the varied leaves of creation, demonstrating the wisdom, the power and the goodness of God, who has given immortality to men.

Are You Really Clean?

The advantages of thorough personal cleanliness are only appreciated by a few, for most people are ignorant of what thorough personal cleanliness means, and consider ablutions which are confined to the face, neck and hands all that is necessary. If one were to say to the average man or woman "You are not clean," it is very certain the average man or woman would be horrified and feel insulted. It is a fact, nevertheless, that largely from ignorance, and partly from prejudice, we go through life "dirty," rarely, if ever, cognizant of the physical pleasure to be derived from perfect cleanliness.

Now, it may be asked here, not inopportunely, "What is perfect cleanliness?" Briefly, let us describe it as that condition which enables the body to breathe with regularity and ease through the pores of the skin. Whenever the body cannot so breathe, we are not clean, and some internal disorder, more or less severe, is the inevitable result. A great many people are sick simply because they are dirty. Cleanliness, as it is generally understood, means that the surface of the skin is free from dirt. This, however, is not real cleanliness. To be really clean, not only the surface of the skin, but its pores, must be free from dirt; furthermore, the blood itself should be free from impurities.

It may be said with truth that dirt on the surface of the skin is not nearly so deleterious as dirt in the pores. This statement is proved by the fact that workmen engaged in labor where proper perspiration is induced, are rarely unhealthy, simply because, though dirty in the ordinary sense of the term, the pores of the skin are kept constantly washed and clean.

Of this fact most of us are ignorant. Our ancestors in olden times were not so ignorant, and knowing full well that hot and cold water washed the skin, but not its pores, in order to keep themselves perfectly clean, used the Hot Air Bath.—*From Food and Health*.

THE BATH IN COLD, ROUGH WEATHER.

There is no luxury on earth that compares with the Hot Air Bath in cold, stormy weather, with the thermometer below zero : the hot rooms may truly be called a paradise on earth. Oh, yes, we hear you say, but how is it when you go out? it must be very dangerous—we shall get cold—I wouldn't take one for a thousand dollars ! Now we assure our readers—those not having the experience—that they are laboring under a delusion, and we regret to say that many who ought to be more truthful, encourage that sort of belief when consulted on the subject. If such was the case, the Bath would fall of its own weight—'twould die out—but twelve year's experience in administering the bath shows that during the winter of each year, the business is *fully one-third* more than in the summer months. Practical knowledge is of much more worth than all theories, or the opinions of those who *think* they know all about it.

A lady writer in Dr. Shepard's neat little quarterly, *The Hammam*, among other good things in relation to the Turkish Bath for ladies, says : "On one point in particular I wish to remove any wrong impression. There is no *exposure* here of beauties, or defects either, not ordinarily visible. 'How nice this is,' said a lady to me one day at the bath; " I thought one was so shockingly exposed.' She found she had a little room to herself where she could undress and wrap a sheet around her, only face and feet being seen, and thus enjoy a luxury which is nowhere to be had except at the Turkish Bath.

There is no royal cure by drugs, rest assured—*no third person in the shape of an atonement.* Nature is run upon the European plan—you get precisely what you pay for, and you pay the debt to the uttermost farthing; nature demands good money; you must either pay, or settle the bill with much suffering.

" Perhaps nothing will so much hasten the time," says Spencer, " when body and mind will both be adequately cared for, as a diffusion of the belief that the preservation of health is a *duty.* Few seem conscious that there is such a thing as *physical morality.* Men's habitual words and acts imply the idea that they are at liberty to treat their bodies as they please. Disorders entailed by disobedience to nature's dictates, they regard simply as grievances, not as the effects of a conduct more or less flagitious. Though the evil consequences inflicted on their dependents and on future generations, are often as great as those caused by crime, yet they do not think themselves in any degree criminal. It is true that, in the case of drunkenness, the viciousness of purely bodily transgression is recognized; but none appear to infer that if this bodily transgression is vicious, so, too, is every bodily transgression. The fact is, *all breaches of the laws of health are physical sins.*"

Real force and primary success fall to the lot of very few men, but sustained perseverance can be practiced by the most humble and insignificant, while its silent power will be found to grow irresistible with time. Fate itself cannot withstand diligence and skill. It is not strength, but perseverance, that wins the battle; and even in social life, it is rather persistency than talents, that wins the coveted prize.

The Turkish Bath should not be considered in the light of a private enterprise. To place the greatest luxury—the most efficient preventive of disease, and the most powerful remedial agent known—within reach of the people, should be treated as one of the *great public questions of the day*, and those who promote it should be regarded as public benefactors, and humanitarians of the first water.

If there is any difference there is greater necessity for the employment of hot air, electric, and Roman baths for ladies than for gentlemen. Indoor life and little exercise cause, in many instances, mental depression, impairment, and physical prostration, with extreme sensibility to climatic changes. They have only to employ these sanitary agents to become healthy, ornamental and useful. They should be early taught the important truth that beauty and health are inseparable, and that both are as certain to follow obedience to organic law as disease is to follow transgression.

In the physical world so long as nature is hurrying the system onward to a perfectly healthy tone, the wise physician will watch, but let nature have its way—while the unwise will dose and blister and purge, reduce, then try to tone up, until the machine is broken down by injudicious experimenting. All persons who attempt to control governments and regulate the public finances should remember that there are certain laws of demand and supply that cannot be contravened without a shock.

———————

" In his diseases Asa sought not to the Lord, but to the physician. And Asa slept with his fathers."

———————

The Bath now stands upon its own merits, a great natural and acknowledged power, and its glory is that like truth, it can enter into no dishonest compromise with error. Let it not, however, be supposed for a moment that we represent the Bath as a Catholican or Panacea: far from it. These is not in nature any sovereign remedy for all diseases, save the avoidance of their causes, but this, at least, is certain, that as far as the unerring evidence of enlightened and verified experience warrants a decided conviction, and justifies its candid expression, the Bath can be most advantageously employed in all diseases: and that, in cases where its curative properties are rendered inoperative by organic disease, it is capable of exercising a most salutary and soothing influence as a demulcent, in abating the virulence of morbid action, and alleviating, *as nothing else can do* the misery of human suffering. *To this extent, and no further, the use of the Bath is advocated.*

Prof. H. von Zeimssen of Munich, Bavaria, in his new Medical Cyclopædia, which has been republished in England and in this country, as a standard work, endorses the hot-air bath—the so-called Turkish Bath, (or Thermæ), and in volume fifteen, on kidney diseases, and especially in nearly all forms of Bright's Disease, after presenting the various remedies which have been relied upon, and which he says are not reliable, he comes to the conclusion that in his opinion, " diaphoresis constitutes the most reliable means of reducing the troublesome and dangerous dropsy."

" It is also the only treatment from which I believe myself justified in expecting a curative action on the process of disease in the kidneys.

" In this sense, an efficient diaphoretic treatment fulfils not only the *indicatio symtomatica*, but actually also the *indicatio-morbi* in a better and surer manner than any other mode of treatment.

" In chronic parynchymatous nephretis also I have repeatedly found, after the adoption of a methodical diaphoretic treatment, that as soon as I succeeded in producing a profuse sweat every day, a more abundant flow of urine set in, and the percentage of albumen became less. We must remember that in the chronic form of the disease, (Bright's Disease), we have to deal with a much more extensive alteration, both of the vessels and the tissues, and if we expect to effect a cure by diaphoresis we must set to work in a thoroughly methodical manner, and carry out the treatment with obstinate pertinacity."

The method most agreeable to the patient, and at the same time, as I believe, most effectual, is to heat the skin by dry hot air, as is done in the so-called Turkish Bath; this plan is greatly to be preferred to vapor baths or sweating closets; this undoubtedly offers the opportunity for producing the longest sweating without any prejudicial effects upon the patient.

"The employment of steam and water baths unavoidably induces considerable elevation of the temperature of the whole body; this cannot be endured for more than a short time without injury. No similar overheating need be induced in hot-air baths, and we should therefore be able to allow our patients to sweat for much longer periods without anxiety.

"It would be at once simplest and most convenient to let these patients take their baths in complete establishments, with comfortable bath rooms, but to meet special contingencies, we could avail ourselves of makeshifts, so called sweating closets, or sand baths, etc."

Excuse me also for calling your attention to a recent statement of Dr. Wallaston, Medical Director of the British army:

"In my professional attendance on the sick, in the hospital at Scutari, I contracted a severe fever, which nearly proved fatal. After having partially recovered, by the skill and zeal of my medical friends, Dr. Delmege and Dr. Calder, of the 47th Regiment, whose names I cannot forbear mentioning, I was induced to try a Turkish Bath, *notwithstanding my debility*. I labored under severe hepatic disease and jaundice, followed by œdema of the legs and abdominal dropsy.

"I confess the first Turkish Bath was somewhat difficult to bear, owing to the exhaustion which attended my illness. Afterwards I greatly enjoyed the Bath, and *each successive one made me feel fresher and fresher, till they materially altered the whole character of my illness.* The copious perspiration gave me immense relief. My skin, which had been hot, dry, parched up, and irritable, now became cool, soft, and pleasant, the cuticle peeled off the whole body like the desquamation from scarlet fever; I had the pleasure of renewing the whole surface of the body, as if I had been moulting The new cuticle was as smooth as velvet, and the organ of touch extremely sensitive, but not at all painful. The biliary secretions gradually returned, the absorbent system, heightened into action, removed the dropsy from the abdomen and extremities, and the general functions improved; I slept better, and my appetite became keen. *I will venture to assert most distinctly that I experienced more benefit from a continuance of the Bath than I derived from all other medicines put together, and that I owe my life to the Turkish Bath.*

———

That the editor of this diminutive sheet has been in St. Louis nearly five years and has never knowingly taken a dose of quinine during his stay; has never had a chill or suffered more than temporary inconvenience from malarial influence, and his simple preventive has been the Turkish Bath. It is simply astonishing to see the amount and quality of ignorance that prevails among intelligent people respecting the Bath. Many believe it to be foretaste of purgatory: a remedy whose possible advantages are more than balanced by the severity of its administration. Never was a greater mistake. If you are worn out by continued labor of

brain or body, if you have a nervous or a bilious head-
ache, if you are troubled with the premonitory symptoms of diarrhœa, do not dose yourself with brandy,
peppermint or opium, take a Turkish Bath; you not
only have the satisfaction of being cured, but of being
cured on sound physiological principles.—*Church of
the Messiah.*

Never was there a greater mistake made than that
perspiration is weakening. It drains away no living
tissue, but merely effete and poisonous matter, which
was oppressing, and not maintaining life. It has become
a question with me, not what the Bath will cure, but
what it will not cure.—*Dr. Brereton, introducer of the
Bath into Australia.*

The Director of the large Bath in Dublin, says:
"In four years we have had one hundred and fifty
thousand bathers. I have never yet known of a person being injured by a bath. I have sometimes heard
reports of injury, but when I have inquired into such
cases, I have invariably found them to be without
foundation."

Persons of sedentary habits, merchants, bankers,
lawyers, ministers, literary men, clerks, men of leisure,
and gentlemen and ladies of wealth and ease, should
take these baths every week as a means of preserving
their health, and thus enhancing all the enjoyments
of life.

The Turkish Bath is peculiarly adapted to ladies.
From their sedentary habits, the circulation of the
blood in the extremities and at the surface is defective.

causing much unpleasantness of feeling, coldness of extremities, torpidity of the skin, sick headache, etc. The Turkish Bath is admirably adapted to relieve this condition, and is destined to be largely used by the ladies, wherever erected. Their effect in beautifying the complexion, improving the health of the skin, and imparting a healthy tone to the body, is truly remarkable.

Every physician knows, though metaphysicians know little about it, that the laws that govern the animal machine are as certain and invariable as those which guide the planetary system, and are as little subject to the control of the human being who is subject to them.

In the reign of Antoninus Caracalla, A. D. 302, Gibbon says: "The baths of Caracalla were opened at stated hours for the indiscriminate service of the senators and the people; that they contained about 1,600 seats of marble, and that the Thermæ could accommodate more than 3,000 persons at one time. They occupied the 'Aventine Mount,' and excelled in beauty, grandeur and extent those of any former Emperor. The whole enclosed space was more than one mile in circumference; the total length of the Thermæ, or hot air chamber, was 1,840 feet, and its breadth 1,476 feet. At each end were two temples; one, dedicated to Appollo, the other, to Æsculapius, as the tutelary deities of a place sacred to the improvement of the mind and health.

"The baths of Diocletian excelled even those of Caracalla in extent and splendor, and were the largest in Rome, or, indeed, in the world, for they were capable of accommodating 18,000 bathers at once.

According to Eusebius, they were completed A. D. 302, and were built, principally, by the enforced labor of Christians, during the tenth and last persecution."

All the baths of the Emperors had the air heated by flues underneath the floor—the hypocaustium—after the Greek model. So highly valued was the bath by the military authorities, as a sanitary institution, that wherever a permanent Roman camp was formed, there, also, baths were constructed to protect the health of the soldiers. The extensive remains of several such have been discovered in England, at London, Chester, Weaxeter, and elsewhere.

SLEEP'S TIME.

Sleep obtained two hours before midnight, when the negative forces are in operation, is the rest which most recuperates the system, giving brightness to the eye and a glow to the cheek. The difference in the appearance of a person who habitually retires at ten o'clock and that of one who sits up until twelve is quite remarkable. The tone of the system, so evident in the complexion, the clearness and sparkle of the eye, and the softness of the lines of the features, is, in a person of health, kept at "concert pitch" by taking regular rest two hours before twelve o'clock, and thereby obtaining the "beauty sleep" of night. There is a heaviness of the eye, a sallowness of the skin, and an absence of that glow in the face which renders it fresh in expression and round in appearance, that readily distinguishes the person who keeps late hours.

AFTER THE BATH.

There comes a dreamy languor o'er me stealing,
  A lassitude which is not lack of strength,
A pulsing rest, a plenitude of feeling,
  Which thrills divinely through my sheeted length.
There's no negation in the soft enjoyment;
  It is not enervation, but delight.
Body and mind find sensuous employment
  In idle shifting and in fancies bright.

Nothing disturbs the self-possessed sensation,
  Each muscle is reliant, and each nerve;
There is an equipoise, a co-relation,
  A perfect balance which they all preserve.
I watch the smoke-wreaths from my lips uprising,
  I note the fountain idling with its spray,
Luxurious adjuncts to a fair devising,
  And lazily the moments pass away.

Such glowing rest might follow a potation
  Of liquor spiced, or still decanted wine,
But so could never come the clean equation
  'Twixt brain and body which I feel in mine.
There is no thought of yet-to-come reaction,
  No forfeit for the passing pleasure's sum,
Here only is a perfect satisfaction
  Of what is present and is yet to come.

Beyond all pale of pleasure apathetic
  He passes who pursues this pleasant path,
A finer zest is his, a thrill magnetic,
  The perfect sequel to the perfect bath.
Nothing is needed the delight enhancing,
  The blood is free in artery and in vein,
'Tis but to will the act to set it dancing
  In turbulent and bubbling course again.

Like tiger basking in the noon-day splendid,
  With nerves relaxed, but still with nerves of steel,
I lie supine 'till the siesta's ended,
  Quiescent, still the tiger's vigor feel;
And then I shake me, like the tiger waking,
  And face the struggles of the day once more,
To laugh at troubles which had set me quaking—
  Mere trifles now which heavy were before.

S. WATERLOO.

St. Louis, Mo., June 11, 1876.

THE BATH CODE.

RULES FOR ITS SAFE AND SALUTARY ADMINISTRATION.

1. Calm and repose of body and mind is the first essential rule of conduct in the bath. All distracting thoughts and passions, therefore, should be left at the door. Even to talk is more or less to excite the brain, and should be avoided as much as possible. The reason of this rule is obvious, because the object sought is to summon into vigorous exercise the more organic or vegetative powers of the economy—to promote for the time the quickened activity of circulation, exhalation, excretion, absorption, etc., and to set at rest the jaded or worried animal nervous system. In other words, to quiet the brain, to soothe the sensitive nerves, and to rouse the organic or nutritive nerves. I verily believe that a large majority of my bathers lose almost, and altogether, the good effects of the bath, by reading in the hot rooms, by discussing exciting subjects, and walking rapidly up and down the rooms while taking their baths.

The diaphoresis, or perspiration, is intended to be brought about, while the bather is in a passive state, it is then *never weakening*, no vital energy is lost. But by tramping, " or go as you please," by working ones self into fever heat, by rubbing your arms and legs to see what discoveries can be made, or talking, thereby inviting the blood to the brain, the bath is lost to all who indulge in such nonsense, aye, worse than lost, for actual injury is done.

2. In cold weather, bathers going in with cold feet, so cold that they almost feel that no fire can warm them, have the first cup of comfort, so to speak, by placing their feet upon a hot tile floor, (far preferable to a hot water foot bath) the feet are soon warmed, and the determination of blood to the head which some bathers complain of (or fear they will have) will be prevented, and perspiration will be induced in a much shorter time.

3. If the uninitiated bather (especially if an invalid, where the skin is inactive) does not perspire readily in fifteen or twenty minutes, he should be taken to the shampooing room and be sponged off thoroughly with warm water, or what is much better, have his or her shampoo there and then, and return to the hot room. If the skin does not act then in a few minutes, the bather should be taken by the attendant back to the shampooing room, cooled off, and sent to cooling room for rest and quiet. The second bath, if taken within a few days after the first one, will be more satisfactory, as free perspiration will be the result after a short time in the hot room. The *supposed case*, above mentioned, very seldom occurs.

4. The time to be spent in the tepid, or hot room, will vary according to the sensation and power of tolerance of the bather; no rule can possibly be laid down for all. As a general rule, however, it is safe to say that from twenty minutes to one hour is a good average for most people. The *skinbound* require longer time than those whose skin acts promptly, but the for-

mer cannot enjoy the bath as well as the latter, consequently, they must not attempt to take too long baths at the commencement of the course.

5. On entering the shampooing room, first in order is to have the shampooing table *warm*, or *hot even*. No one should allow themselves to lie down upon a cold, or even a cool slab; (better ten times go without your shampoo, however much you may enjoy the *manipulator's gentle touch*); for a cold is sure to follow such a perversion of what a Turkish Bath should be.

6. To get the tonic or stimulating effect of the bath the attendant should work rapidly and vigorously, (not roughly, by any means); let the manipulations be quiet and gentle; use warm water freely for cleansing the body from soap; then cool, followed by cold, for a *few seconds*. In cold weather the time occupied in spraying off and cooling should not be *more than two minutes*, then the bather gets the tonic and stimulating effects of a Turkish Bath. On the contrary, if the bather allows the attendant to spray him for five or ten minutes, as many do, it takes the electricity all out of a person, and utterly destroys the good effects of a proper bath. A man is not a fish, and cannot flourish and grow strong under such treatment, however pleasant it may be to the bather.

7. The skin is best allowed to dry in a warm sheet, while taking rest on the couch in the cooling room. Very little rubbing should be done with towels, as the skin is very sensitive and delicate after a Turkish bath. The time spent in the cooling room—the luxurious time of the bath—may be from fifteen minutes to a half hour, or longer if desired.

8. The bath should never be taken on a full stomach; two hours should certainly intervene after a heavy dinner.

9 There are cases—a feeble person, or one suffering from a severe cold—when, after entering the cooling room, or when about to dress, feel a little chilly. Such a one should enter the hot room for a few moments, take a turn up and down the room ; the chilly feeling will at once subside, and will not return.

10. When the object is to deplete or disgorge congested organs, (as the liver, spleen, or the kidneys), then the profuse perspiration, at the sole expense of the existing fluids in the body, will be more likely to drain off the excess of blood from the overloaded organ. To this end, withhold all fluids during the process, excepting perhaps in some cases of kidney disease

If the above advice would be followed by the patrons of a bath, much more good would be derived therefrom, and better results attained.

Proper advice *by a physician is well*, but not prescribed at random, or to be invoked at the beck or whim of every patron who has once or twice experienced its solaces. I happen to know that already the bath, like all other good things, is being abused ; especially in this, where old bathers volunteer their advice to new bathers, and especially so where the bather is an invalid.

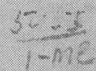

Made in the USA
Middletown, DE
16 December 2017